Run Your Mind
Training Workbook

JULIA RAFFAINI

Copyright © 2019 Julia Raffaini

All rights reserved.

ISBN: 9781793032904

DEDICATION

This book is dedicated to my amazing husband. Thank you for continuing to support me on my running journey and for encouraging me to write this workbook.

CONTENTS

1 INTRODUCTION 1

2 GOAL DEVELOPMENT 20

3 MENTAL TOUGHNESS 45

4 CONFIDENCE 56

5 CONCENTRATION 63

6 ENERGY MANAGEMENT 99

7 CARING FOR THE BODY 108

8 TRAINING JOURNAL 125

9 SAMPLE TRAINING PLANS 198

WORKSHEETS

1	THOUGHTS/ FEELINGS	3
2	ABC	8
3	COGNITIVE DISTORTION	15
4	VALUES	28
5	PROS/ CONS	65
6	MINDFULNESS SCHEDULE	66
7	MINDFULNESS TRACKING	67
8	ABC	76
9	CHANGING EMOTIONS	84
10	SELF-CRITICISM	92

ACKNOWLEDGMENTS

I want to begin by thanking my husband, Michael Raffaini, for encouraging me to create this workbook and for being one of my editors. I'm grateful for his support through my running training and racing over the years. He has trained with me and has been my race support many times including, but not limited to, providing early morning transportation to race starts, fuel and hydration support, and words of encouragement. I would also like to thank him for supporting me in completing the personal training certification program at the National Academy of Sports Medicine and the running training certification program at Run-Fit. This training has given me a solid foundation to build from in supporting myself and others through running and fitness.

Next, I would like to thank my mom, Amy Cooper, for being one of my editors and for her collaboration in developing the yoga routines in this book. Providing yoga training for the past 30+ years, she continues to be an inspiration in the fitness/health industry. I want to thank her for her Yoga Teacher Training program through the Shasta Yoga Institute which I was blessed to be able to complete in 2014. This yoga training has helped to support my health and running for many years.

Finally, I would like to thank my first running coach, David Clark, for his guidance. He is an inspiring athlete and provided me with a great coaching experience.

1 INTRODUCTION

Are you a new runner looking to make the most of your running experience? Are you a seasoned runner looking to improve your performance? Have you hit a plateau in your training? Have you noticed your motivation and love of running waning?

Sport psychology refers to the application of psychological techniques and principles in sports. This is a newer field in psychology and can be vital to a runner's success. One could argue that training the mind is just as important if not more important than training the body in sports performance. Sport psychology can address a wide variety of challenges impacting training and performance including motivation, goal development, mental toughness, concentration, confidence, mental imagery, and energy management.

Navigating this workbook

In this workbook, I focus on introducing you to psychological principles and techniques to utilize to improve your running training and performance. I use reflective questions and activities designed to help you to quickly and easily begin implementing these techniques. These techniques can support a wide array of growth such as helping you to move out of a plateau in your training, helping you to perform better on race day, and helping you to get more out of your training sessions currently.

In Chapters 1 through 6, the information provided is focused on psychological principals, goal development, mental toughness, confidence, concentration, and energy management. As you continue past Chapter 6, you will find a section that addresses caring for the body which includes a couple of yoga routines that you can utilize to supplement your running training. Next, you will find a training journal section. This section is designed to help you to integrate what you have learned in the previous chapters into your running training. While some runners may choose to use this journal while they read this book, others may want to complete the rest of the workbook before starting to use the journal section. Please use this journal in whatever manner you feel is most useful to you. Finally, while this workbook is not meant to take the place of a training plan, I have included some sample plans for you to utilize if you desire. These sample plans can be found in Chapter 9. Please keep in mind that it is ideal to follow a training plan that has been custom made to address your fitness level and goals.

Understanding how thoughts affect feelings & behaviors

Before moving into some of the main concepts in sport psychology, let's begin by discussing how thoughts affect feelings and behaviors. Cognitive behavioral therapy teaches us that our feelings and behaviors are a result of how we are thinking. Below are three examples of how someone could respond differently to the same situation based on their thoughts:

- Scenario number one: Jim's boss tells him that he is fired. Jim thinks "yes, I've wanted to leave this job for a year and now I can move on to a new job with the support of receiving unemployment between jobs. Maybe this is an opportunity for me to pursue job training." Jim feels happy and thanks his boss for the opportunity.

- Scenario number two: Jim's boss tells him that he's fired. Jim thinks "well, I have liked this job and I wish that I wasn't being fired. However, it's not the end of the world and maybe my next job will be just as enjoyable." Jim feels calm and thanks his boss for the opportunity before inquiring if there is any room for him to improve and keep his current job.

- Scenario number three: Jim's boss tells him that he's fired. Jim thinks "I cannot believe this terrible thing is happening. I need this job, and I am a failure." Jim becomes upset and yells at his boss before storming out of the office.

We all have developed patterns of thinking based on our experiences. Some of our assumptions and beliefs can be unhelpful leading to poor performance and dysfunction. By examining our thoughts, we can create effective and lasting change in our behaviors/ performance. To do that, let's first distinguish a thought from a feeling.

Thoughts:	Feelings:
I think…	I feel…
I can't be successful	Hopeless, sad
I won't be happy ever again	Hopeless, depressed
I am a terrible runner	Sad, depressed
I worked hard during training	Proud, happy

To practice distinguishing between thoughts and feelings and to begin tracking your thoughts and feelings, please utilize the following worksheet this week. While this worksheet can be useful to apply to thoughts and feelings related to training immediately, it is also very helpful to use in your life beyond your running training. The more that you practice using this worksheet, the easier and quicker it will be to identify your thoughts and feelings.

Thoughts/ Feelings Worksheet:

Thoughts	Feelings

Thoughts	Feelings

Thoughts	Feelings

Thoughts	Feelings

Thoughts	Feelings

Now that you have had the opportunity to practice identifying thoughts and feelings, let's move on to using a more common format to track and examine thoughts and feelings. The next worksheet includes a section to support you in practicing disputing your thoughts and replacing unhelpful/inaccurate thoughts.

ABC Worksheet:

Activating event (What happened?)	Belief (What did you say to yourself?)	Consequence (What did you feel? What did you do?)

Was your belief reasonable? Was it based in fact? What evidence supports this?	In the future, what could you say to yourself instead?

Activating event (What happened?)	Belief (What did you say to yourself?)	Consequence (What did you feel? What did you do?)

Was your belief reasonable? Was it based in fact? What evidence supports this?	In the future, what could you say to yourself instead?

Activating event (What happened?)	Belief (What did you say to yourself?)	Consequence (What did you feel? What did you do?)

Was your belief reasonable? Was it based in fact? What evidence supports this?	In the future, what could you say to yourself instead?

Remember how I said that we all have developed patterns of thinking based on our experiences? And that sometimes these beliefs and assumptions lead to poor performance and dysfunction? In cognitive behavioral therapy, there is a list of cognitive distortions or thinking errors that many people experience. Below I have provided a summary of these common cognitive distortions to help you identify your unhelpful thinking patterns.

Cognitive distortions

Cognitive distortions are distortions in thinking. Everyone experiences cognitive distortions from time to time. Being able to identify and label them is the first step towards correcting this erroneous thinking. Before practicing identification of cognitive distortions in the Cognitive Distortion Worksheet below, familiarize yourself with the following common cognitive distortions:

1. Fortune telling: predicting the future.

2. Mind reading: assuming what others are thinking.

3. Discounting positives: not recognizing and/or minimizing positives.

4. Labeling: assigning broad negative traits.

5. Negative filter: focusing on the negatives while not noticing the positives.

6. Dichotomous thinking: viewing things as all-or-nothing. Example: "everyone hates me."

7. Overgeneralizing: believing in blanket negative patterns based on a single incident. Example: after being unsuccessful once, saying "I usually fail."

8. Shoulds: instead of being in the moment with what is, making statements about what should or shouldn't be.

9. Blaming: rather than taking personal responsibility, blaming others.

10. Personalizing: rather than acknowledging others' roles, assigning an unreasonable amount of blame on yourself.

11. Unfair comparisons: judging yourself and setting unrealistic expectations for yourself based on comparisons to others.

12. What if: a series of "what if" statements yielding unsatisfying answers.

13. Emotional reasoning: allowing your emotions to dictate your interpretation of reality.

14. Regret orientation: focusing on what you could have done differently in the past.

15. Judgment focus: utilizing black and white evaluations to judge yourself, others, and events

16. Inability to disconfirm: disregarding or rejecting any information that contradicts your negative thoughts.

17. Catastrophizing: believing that something is or will be so terrible that you will not be able to withstand it.

Cognitive Distortion Worksheet:

Thought	Feeling	Cognitive distortion

Thought	Feeling	Cognitive distortion

Thought	Feeling	Cognitive distortion

Thought	Feeling	Cognitive distortion

Thought	Feeling	Cognitive distortion

2 GOAL DEVELOPMENT

Your alarm goes off at 5 a.m. It's dark outside, and you can hear the rain bouncing off the roof of your house. You had intended to run this morning, but your bed is just so comfortable and warm. You start thinking: "would it really hurt to miss this one run? I can just push a little harder during my run tomorrow." Excuses continue to flood your mind. What is it that gets you out of bed and lacing up your running shoes? What is the source of your motivation? For most runners, this is where goal setting comes into play. This chapter will focus on helping you to establish effective goals and to work with your motivation.

What are your running goals? Establishing both long-term and short-term goals are ideal.

Examples of running goals include:

- I want to run a 5K PR
- I want to complete a marathon
- I want to feel more prepared on race day
- I want to feel more confident as a runner
- I want to run 5 days per week
- I want to reduce my racing anxiety
- I want to run with friends more often.

Select two to three goals to focus on. Please write these goals in the space below:

Take a moment to consider how you can make these goals more specific and, if they are not yet measurable, take a moment to make them measurable.

Set deadlines for your goals and break down the steps you will need to take to reach these goals.

Finally, write down why you have selected these goals? What is motivating you?

Look at your schedule and identify where your running training will fit into your current schedule. How does you current schedule need to change? Consider times of the day that you feel more energetic and also consider training times in relation to meal times.

What obstacles do you think may interfere with your training?

What can you do to mitigate these obstacles?

Developing SMART goals

When developing your goals, use SMART goals. SMART stands for Specific, Measurable, Attainable, Relevant, and Timely.
Looking at the goals you developed in this chapter, see if you can improve your goals a little more by asking yourself the following:

1. Are my goals specific?

2. Are my goals measurable? In other works, how can I see/document my progress towards these goals?

3. Are these goals attainable?

4. Are they relevant? Why are they important? Do they relate to other goals?

5. Are they timely? Have I set deadlines for myself to reach these goals?

Bonus activity

Share your goals with someone else. Sharing goals can help you to become more accountable as well as to develop a stronger support system.

Motivation

There are three kinds of motivation: internal, external, and amotivation. It is essential to understand these three types in order to optimally work with your motivation to improve your training and performance. External motivation refers to motivation that is fueled by external rewards or rewards outside yourself such as winning money at a race. Internal motivation refers to the kind of motivation that comes from within such as when someone engages in a sport for the joy of it. Amotivation refers to a lack of motivation. While motivation can naturally fluctuate, you can work to increase your motivation using sport psychology. While internal motivation is vital for long term running success, external motivation can be very effective when paired with internal motivation. External motivation can be especially useful for short term goals and can help to motivate you as you work towards long term goals as well. You can create your reinforcement by building in external rewards to fuel your training. For example, you could develop a plan to reward yourself with a special drink after your long run.

Problem solving your motivation

When motivation wanes, the first step to working with your motivation is to identify why there has been a shift. Sometimes a decrease in motivation is related to decreased confidence, poor health, fatigue/inadequate recovery, and burnout. Addressing these specific challenges will be important as well as spending some time getting in touch with your internal motivation for running. For information about working with confidence and physical health: We will focus on confidence in Chapter 4 and caring for the body in Chapter 7.

Burn out

It is normal for a runner to feel burnt out from time to time. Training is challenging, and it's normal for athletes to need a break to regain perspective and fall back in love with running. Sometimes this break means just taking a few days off of running and doing something different such as swimming or biking. Doing different forms of exercise provides valuable cross-training while allowing recovery from burnout. However, sometimes a runner needs to take more time off to find balance and care for their physical and mental needs. Taking this time off is valuable in order to return to training stronger and is part of your running training. Perhaps training at this time means focusing on building your coping skills. Maybe it is time to taking a closer look at how you are prioritizing and how you are utilizing time management strategies.

If you find that you are repeatedly having challenges with motivation, perhaps it's time to reevaluate your goals. Sometimes people have challenges with motivation when they are focused more on goals related to ego as opposed to goals related to achieving specific tasks.

Many runners benefit from monitoring their motivation regularly. Please use the questions below to check in with yourself as frequently as is helpful in order to monitor and work with your motivation.

What currently motivates you to run? Identify your internal motivation and external motivation.

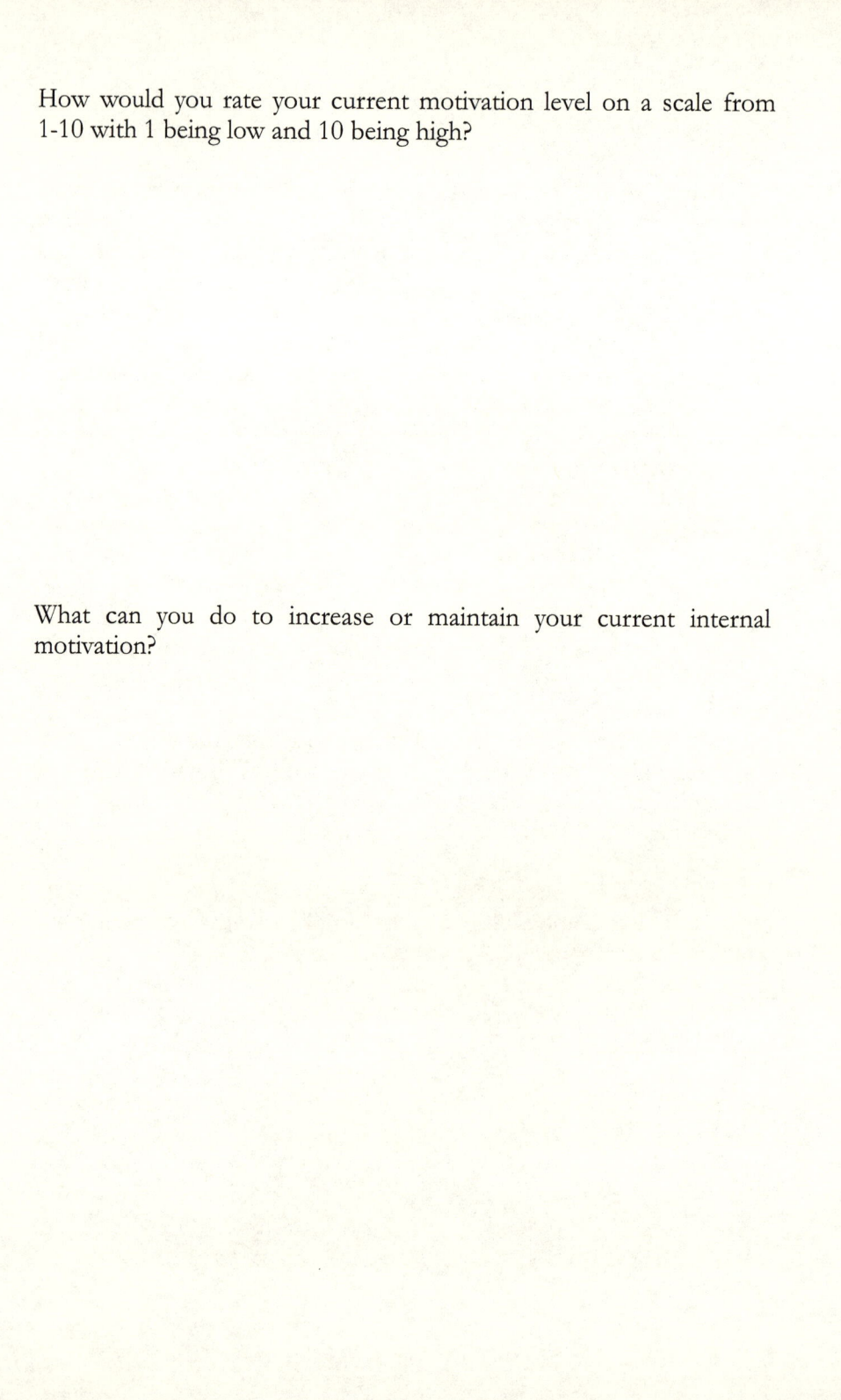

How would you rate your current motivation level on a scale from 1-10 with 1 being low and 10 being high?

What can you do to increase or maintain your current internal motivation?

What can you do to increase or maintain your current external motivation?

Reevaluating priorities & time management strategies

At one point or another, all of us need to reevaluate our priorities and time management strategies. I have found that an excellent first step is to examine values.

In the following activity, please review all of the values before ranking your top 20 by rating 1-20 (1=most important & 20=least important) next to the values on the chart. For these top 20, please answer the questions in the columns next to the value column. I recommend beginning this activity by circling the values that are important to you before going through the process of ranking them. You will notice that some of the values seem similar to one another and this is intentional. Each value has a slightly different meaning to each of us. Consider these differences before selecting your top values. Make sure that you have adequate time for this activity as it can be lengthy.

Values Worksheet:

Values	How do you currently pursue these values?	For those values that are especially important to you, how can you pursue them more often or more effectively in the future?
Wisdom		
Wealth		
Achievement		
Spirituality		
Success		
Trustworthiness		
Stability		
Statuts		
Service		
Security		

Values	How do you currently pursue these values?	For those values that are especially important to you, how can you pursue them more often or more effectively in the future?
Leadership		
Learning		
Loyalty		
Humor		
Happiness		
Kindness		
Knowledge		
Justice		
Influence		
Honesty		

Values	How do you currently pursue these values?	For those values that are especially important to you, how can you pursue them more often or more effectively in the future?
Growth		
Competency		
Creativity		
Curiosity		
Determination		
Fairness		
Friendship		
Fun		
Fame		
Contribution		

Values	How do you currently pursue these values?	For those values that are especially important to you, how can you pursue them more often or more effectively in the future?
Community		
Authority		
Autonomy		
Balance		
Boldness		
Beauty		
Compassion		
Challenge		
Citizenship		
Adventure		

Values	How do you currently pursue these values?	For those values that are especially important to you, how can you pursue them more often or more effectively in the future?
Authenticity		
Poise		
Acceptance		
Assertiveness		
Bravery		
Ambition		
Accountability		
Adaptability		
Charity		
Communication		

Values	How do you currently pursue these values?	For those values that are especially important to you, how can you pursue them more often or more effectively in the future?
Commitment		
Concentration		
Comfort		
Consistency		
Contentment		
Control		
Courage		
Discipline		
Endurance		
Empathy		

Values	How do you currently pursue these values?	For those values that are especially important to you, how can you pursue them more often or more effectively in the future?
Equality		
Family		
Focus		
Freedom		
Generosity		
Grace		
Gratitude		
Humility		
Honor		
Intelligence		

Values	How do you currently pursue these values?	For those values that are especially important to you, how can you pursue them more often or more effectively in the future?
Hard work		
Strength		
Talent		
Teamwork		
Thoughtful		
Tranquility		
Unity		
Victory		
Wonder		
Solitude		

Values	How do you currently pursue these values?	For those values that are especially important to you, how can you pursue them more often or more effectively in the future?
Self-reliance		
Selfless		
Simplicity		
Sensitivity		
Spontaneous		
Present		
Productivity		
Purpose		
Quality		
Recognition		
Decisiveness		

Values	How do you currently pursue these values?	For those values that are especially important to you, how can you pursue them more often or more effectively in the future?
Responsibility		
Respect		
Calmness		
Reputation		
Popularity		
Pleasure		
Openness		
Peace		
Love		
Optimism		

Values	How do you currently pursue these values?	For those values that are especially important to you, how can you pursue them more often or more effectively in the future?
Professionalism		
Realistic		
Recreation		
Reverence		
Imagination		
Insightful		
Lawful		
Logic		
Intuitive		
Organization		

Values	How do you currently pursue these values?	For those values that are especially important to you, how can you pursue them more often or more effectively in the future?
Moderation		
Motivation		
Originality		
Patience		
Order		
Persistence		
Power		
Inspiring		
Innovation		
Inquisitive		

Values	How do you currently pursue these values?	For those values that are especially important to you, how can you pursue them more often or more effectively in the future?
Hope		
Health		
Harmony		
Goodness		
Expressiveness		
Other:		
Other:		
Other:		
Other:		
Other:		

How was this activity for you? Was it challenging or easy? How so?

Were you surprised by your value choices? If so, what was surprising?

What do you currently prioritize? How are your top ranking values reflected in this?

In what way, if at all, do you want to shift your priorities to better reflect your values?

What steps do you need to take to make this shift? (Think long term and short term shifts)

How does running fit with your values/ priorities?

General time management strategies

1. Begin the day with focus. Check in with your goals and purpose.

2. Create a task list. Be clear and specific.

3. Prioritize your list by examining which activities are most important and would have the greatest positive impact and which activities are least important and would have the least negative impact if left undone.

4. Create an environment with minimal interruptions.

5. Avoid avoiding. Many of us fall into the trap of avoiding activities we don't want to do. By procrastinating, we are not doing ourselves any favors. If you find yourself in this trap, establish a deadline for yourself to complete the task and plan a small reward that you can earn by completing this task.

6. Schedule time to relax. Whether it be a 5 minute walk or a 10 minute meditation, breaking up your day with relaxing activities can help you maintain better time management.

7. Take time to stay organized.

8. Delegate tasks when possible.

9. Do one activity at a time. Give each task your undivided attention rather than multitasking.

10. At the end of your day, take time to reflect. Review your task list from the day and develop a new list for tomorrow. Focus on your successes today and acknowledge the obstacles that arose. Spend a few minutes developing a plan to minimize any obstacles that could arise tomorrow.

3 MENTAL TOUGHNESS

This chapter will focus on helping you build your mental toughness. Mental toughness refers to the mental strength that allows you to perform well under pressure, maintain concentration and motivation, and bounce back from setbacks. Mental toughness has a relationship with physical fitness as well as confidence. When the body is stronger, we can display more mental toughness in training. Mental toughness training can be emphasized during physical training to increase success. Moreover, as mental toughness rises, confidence naturally rises. Increased confidence allows a runner to worry less and improve concentration.

Assessing mental toughness

How would you rate your mental toughness on a scale from 1-10 with 1 being low and 10 being high?

How do you respond to feedback?

How to you handle yourself after making a mistake?

How do you handle race pressures?

How do you handle being injured or sick?

How do you respond when facing adversity?

How would you rate your certainty that you can accomplish your running goals? Rate yourself on a scale from 1-10 with 1 being low and 10 being high. Why do you rate yourself at this level? What would it look like to be one number higher? What would it look like to be one number lower?

How would you rate the quality of your concentration during training? Rate yourself on a scale from 1-10 with 1 being low and 10 being high. What would it look like to be one number higher? What would it look like to be one number lower?

Practicing mental toughness in all aspects of your life will help you improve your mental toughness in relation to running. Asking others for feedback on how they observe your mental toughness can add valuable insight to utilize when developing a mental toughness training plan.

Developing your mental toughness training plan

After assessing your mental toughness earlier in this chapter, you probably have a good understanding of your current strengths and weaknesses. Feedback from others may have added to this understanding. The questions below can help you assess for weaknesses and strengths that present in your day to day life.

How do you handle challenging tasks at work?

How do you manage challenging relationships at work?

Do you confront or avoid challenging conversations?

How easy is it for you to reach out for support or guidance?

How do you express your feelings? How do you express challenging feelings such as anger?

How do feel about your ability to set boundaries? Rate yourself on a scale from 1-10 with 1 being low and 10 being high. What would it look like to be one number higher? What would it look like to be one number lower?

Identify three situations in or out of training that you utilized mental toughness.

1.

2.

3.

What helped you to demonstrate mental toughness in these instances?

Identify three situations in or out of training that you did NOT utilize mental toughness.

1.

2.

3.

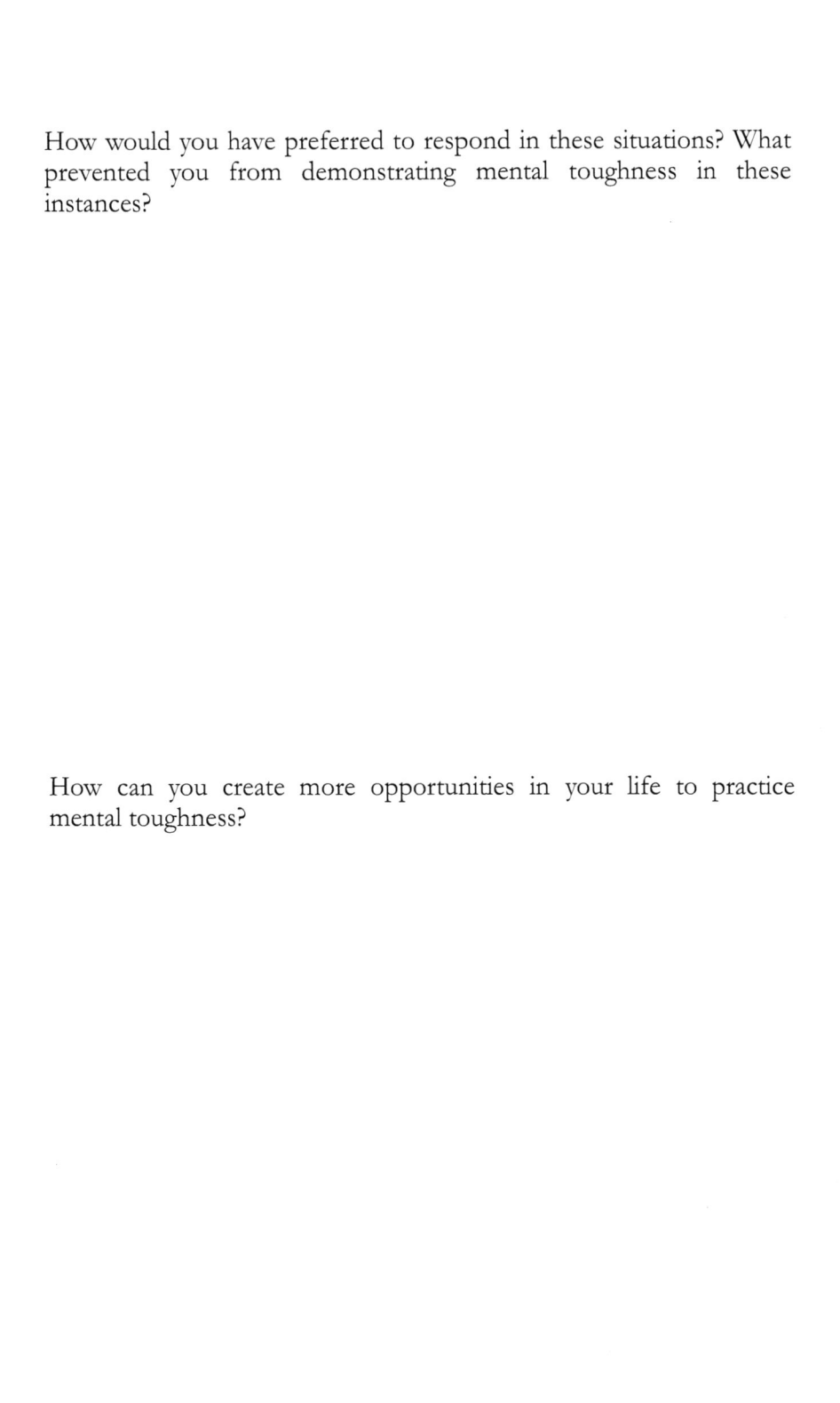

How would you have preferred to respond in these situations? What prevented you from demonstrating mental toughness in these instances?

How can you create more opportunities in your life to practice mental toughness?

What can you do to help yourself successfully demonstrate mental toughness in these activities?

Mental toughness is also related to physical fitness. How can you work to increase your fitness to impact your mental toughness?

Focus on mental toughness in your training and in your life beyond running training this month. Remind yourself of this focus before training and throughout your day. Seek opportunities to practice mental toughness. Rate your success at the end of the day and identify obstacles that prevented you from demonstrating mental toughness when applicable. Share this focus with others in your support system to help yourself remain accountable and ask for continued feedback from those around you.

Bonus activity

There are many books written by runners with great mental toughness. Spend some time with these books…. they can be a great source of inspiration and could provide some additional examples of how you could practice mental toughness.

4 CONFIDENCE

Confidence, or sometimes referred to as self-efficacy, refers to one's belief in one's abilities. As discussed in the previous chapter, increasing mental toughness increases confidence. This chapter will focus on other strategies that runners can use to improve confidence. When a runner is more confident, they often take more risks and can experience more success. Confidence can help a runner to dream big and to be successful in working towards big long-term goals. Runners with higher confidence can benefit from increased effort during training, improved concentration, more positive feelings about training, and increased success overcoming setbacks.

There are several self-efficacy subcategories including scheduling self-efficacy and recovery self-efficacy. Scheduling self-efficacy refers to one's confidence in their ability to goal set and plan for training. Recovery self-efficacy refers to one's belief in their abilities to return to training after a break. Meanwhile, trait-confidence refers to the idea that confidence can be a stable characteristic of one's personality and state-confidence refers to confidence that is dependent on a state of mind and has a shorter duration.

How would you rate your current scheduling self efficacy on a scale from 1-10 with 1 being low and 10 being high?

How would you rate your current recovery self efficacy on a scale from 1-10 with 1 being low and 10 being high?

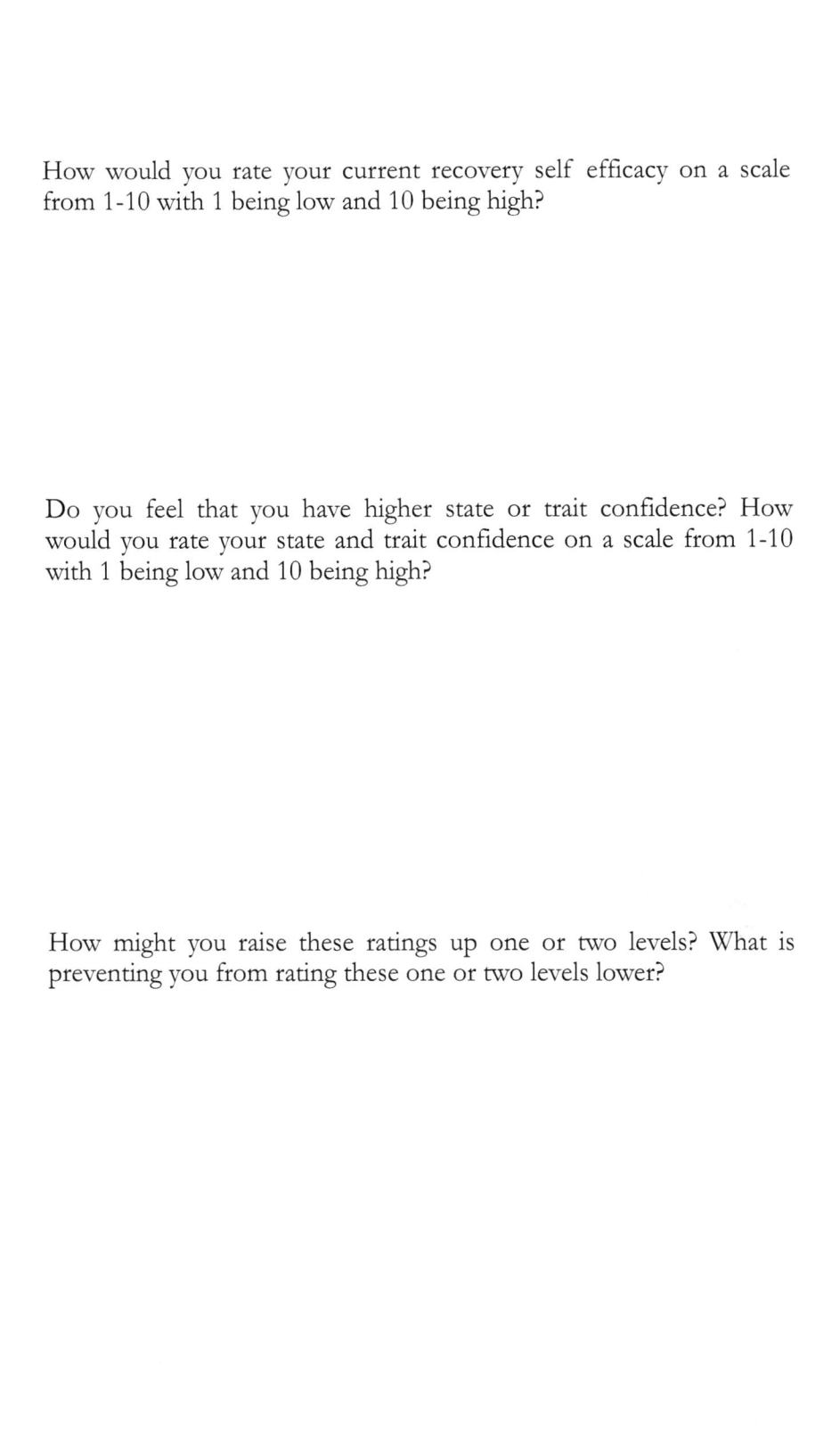

Do you feel that you have higher state or trait confidence? How would you rate your state and trait confidence on a scale from 1-10 with 1 being low and 10 being high?

How might you raise these ratings up one or two levels? What is preventing you from rating these one or two levels lower?

Whenever we experience success, our confidence increases. In other words, when a runner believes that they can get a Boston qualifying time in a marathon, they work hard to reach these goals, and, when they successfully race a Boston qualifying time, then their confidence goes up. Using positive thinking to begin this cycle is a great way to build confidence. As you work through your training plan and you continue to practice positive thinking such as "I can accomplish this run" and "I'm putting in the work to reach these goals," you are actively working to increase your confidence. As you find success in your goals, this confidence will continue to strengthen. Similar to training the body, training the mind can feel uncomfortable and can be challenging. Utilizing positive thinking can feel very strange at first, but with practice, it will feel more natural and will come easier.

Use the following questions to promote confidence in your daily life:

In what ways have you been successful recently?

What helped you be successful?

What can you do to promote your success in the future?

How do you act as your own cheerleader?

What are the words that you say to yourself when you are not feeling confident?

How can you improve upon these statements?

How do you take risks? Are they appropriate and useful risks to help you build success?

Do you track your success effectively?

How do you celebrate your success? How can you improve in this area?

Affirmations

Affirmations are another useful tool to help in building confidence. Affirmations are statements that we say to ourselves that take place in the present moment, are positive, and focus on a specific behavior. Examples of affirmations are "I can complete this Marathon with a 3:30 time" or "I am a fast 5k Runner."

Take a moment to identify several affirmations that you can utilize to improve your confidence. List several that are running specific and several that are related to your daily life outside of training.

1.

2.

3.

4.

5.

6.

Increase confidence through modeling, mastery, social support, and preparation. Modeling refers to learning by observing others. Seeing others successfully working towards their running goals can help a runner build confidence. Runners can find role models by reading running books, participating in social media, or by participating in local running groups. Mastery can be a potent tool to build confidence. Breaking down goals and setting expectations that one can accomplish will help a runner increase confidence over time. Receiving positive feedback and encouragement can serve as another tool to promote confidence. Lastly, both mental and physical preparation is an important factor impacting confidence levels. This can include using imagery (discussed in chapter 5), maintaining concentration (discussed in chapter 5), and caring for the body (discussed in chapter 7).

Additional tips to promote confidence

- To promote confidence building during your training, focus on the journey not the destination. In other words, focus on goals that are about how you are going to reach your goals (ie. how you are training/the process of training).

- Focus on your success every day.

- Take time to check in with your confidence level. Rate your confidence on a scale from 1-10 with 1 being low and 10 being high on a daily basis.

- Focus on skills that are related to mastery rather than ego.

- Recognize and focus on aspects of training that you can control as opposed to those that are not in your power to control.

5 CONCENTRATION

Concentration allows us to work with our body and mind to perform at its best while running. Concentration can function as a spotlight enabling the runner to focus on critical running factors such as stride, self-talk, and motivation while tuning out stimuli that are unimportant for running. Concentration allows us to learn new skills and improve our skills. While there are many distractions both internal and external that threaten to pull a runner's focus away from their sport, there are also numerous techniques that can be used to strengthen one's ability to concentrate. These strategies include meditation, self-monitoring, mindfulness, self-talk, and developing specific routines. This chapter will first discuss the various types of attention and distractions before exploring techniques to improve concentration.

Types of attention include narrow, broad, internal, and external. Narrow attention refers to blocking out all irrelevant cues and focusing only on a couple of cues during a task. Irrelevant cues are all cues that are not relevant to complete the current task. For example, during a run, this would be any other cues beyond completing the task of running. A broad attentional focus refers to receiving many cues to complete the task at hand. Internal attention refers to attention focused inward while external attention refers to attention focused outward.

Runners use both associative and dissociative strategies. Associative strategies involve paying attention to feelings and bodily functions while dissociative strategies involve dissociation from feelings and body sensations such as boredom or pain. Runners may move between these two strategies, but many runners feel that they perform better using associative strategies.

Internal and external distractions include thinking about the past and thinking about the future as well as auditory and visual distractions. Ruminating about the past and worrying about the future are common challenges in and out of training and performance. The following techniques can help a runner mitigate these distractions and improve concentration.

Mindfulness

Mindfulness is the activity of focusing the mind on the present moment without attachments to the moment and without judgment. People are brought to practice mindfulness for many different reasons which include a desire to experience things as they are, to increase happiness and reduce suffering, and to increase mental control.

There are many ways to practice mindfulness. Some of these ways are:

1. Simply noticing the sensations in your body using all of your senses.

2. Observing thoughts that pop into your head before letting them float away like clouds.

3. Observing each feeling that arises without attachment. You can picture them like waves in the ocean ebbing and flowing.

4. Paying attention to the present moment. Noticing what's happening both inside and outside of yourself.

5. Utilizing words to enhance mindfulness by labelling whatever thought or feeling arises (ie. "planning" or "sadness") without judgment. You can notice and label actions. Exclude interpretations and stick just to the fact. Continue to maintain focus on sensations.

6. Focusing completely on the activity you're doing in the present

moment.

7. Focusing on doing one activity at a time.

Mindfulness takes practice. Take a moment to consider and list the pros and/or cons of incorporating a mindfulness practice into your life.

Pros/Cons Worksheet:

PROS	CONS
ie. greater mental control	ie. discomfort from being present with difficult feelings

If you choose to incorporate a mindfulness practice into your life, then commit to a mindfulness training schedule. Indicate which days and times you intend to practice mindfulness. Circle AM or PM or indicate a more specific time.

Mindfulness Schedule:

DAYS	TIMES
Monday	AM PM
Tuesday	AM PM
Wednesday	AM PM
Thursday	AM PM
Friday	AM PM
Saturday	AM PM
Sunday	AM PM

You can utilize the worksheet below to track your mindfulness practices. Rate the quality of your mindfulness after each mindfulness activity on a scale from 1-10. On this scale, 1 refers to challenges being in the present moment/being mindful and 10 refers to feeling focused, centered, and mindful during this activity.

Mindfulness Tracking Worksheet:

DAY	MINDFULNESS ACTIVITY	MINDFULNESS RATING

DAY	MINDFULNESS ACTIVITY	MINDFULNESS RATING

DAY	MINDFULNESS ACTIVITY	MINDFULNESS RATING

DAY	MINDFULNESS ACTIVITY	MINDFULNESS RATING

DAY	MINDFULNESS ACTIVITY	MINDFULNESS RATING

DAY	MINDFULNESS ACTIVITY	MINDFULNESS RATING

Self-monitoring

Self-monitoring is about monitoring oneself. Self-monitoring can involve observing and recording a specific aspect of a runner's life or training plan. This observation strategically directs a runner's attention and can promote mindfulness. Self-monitoring can focus on physical and mental characteristics. Monitoring specific thoughts as well as using tracking devices such as Garmin training watches to track running progress are two examples of the many self-monitoring options.

Self-talk

Self-talk refers to talking to oneself either out loud or silently. We all have self-talk, and it can be both positive and negative. Increasing self-talk that helps a runner let go of inner dialogue about the past or future and return to the present moment will help a runner minimize inner distractions. Examples of self-statements that can be used to help a runner let go of rumination about the past include "There is nothing I can do about the past" and "I did the best I could with the information that I had at the time." Self-talk that can be used to help minimize worries about the future include "Worrying about it won't help" and "I will do my best." Instructional self-talk involves speaking to oneself about how to conduct the task at hand, and this can improve focus on relevant cues and can be effective in mitigating external and internal distractions. Motivational self-talk includes coaching oneself with motivational statements such as "You can do this" and "You have prepared for this."

Do you typically find yourself more distracted by internal or external distractions?

What do you currently do to mitigate these distractions?

What do you find yourself saying to yourself when you realize you are distracted?

How could you improve upon your self-talk to mitigate distractions during running?

Bouncing back

How you bounce back from setbacks and mistakes can have a significant impact on training. When you can quickly bounce back and learn from your experience, you can return to focusing on training right away. When you engage in self-defeating and unproductive self-talk after setbacks and mistakes, it can hold you back.

Negative thoughts are a common obstacle for runners. Utilize the following ABC worksheet introduced in chapter one, to adjust negative thoughts.

ABC Worksheet:

Activating event (What happened?)	Belief (What did you say to yourself?)	Consequence (What did you feel? What did you do?)

Was your belief reasonable? Was it based in fact? What evidence supports this?	In the future, what could you say to yourself instead?

Activating event (What happened?)	Belief (What did you say to yourself?)	Consequence (What did you feel? What did you do?)

Was your belief reasonable? Was it based in fact? What evidence supports this?	In the future, what could you say to yourself instead?

Activating event (What happened?)	Belief (What did you say to yourself?)	Consequence (What did you feel? What did you do?)

Was your belief reasonable? Was it based in fact? What evidence supports this?	In the future, what could you say to yourself instead?

Activating event (What happened?)	Belief (What did you say to yourself?)	Consequence (What did you feel? What did you do?)

Was your belief reasonable? Was it based in fact? What evidence supports this?	In the future, what could you say to yourself instead?

Working with the facts

Examining the facts can help you to identify whether you are reacting to an event and can help you to detect errors in your thinking. This process can also help you to become more aware of your thought patterns and can help you practice identifying cognitive distortions. Utilize the following activity to practice examining facts and experiment with how this activity may be a helpful tool to change emotions.

Changing Emotions Worksheet:

What is the emotion that you want to change?	What event lead to you experiencing this emotion?	Are there any judgements or drastic statements in your description of this event?

What are your interpretations and assumptions about the facts?	What errors can you identify in your interpretations and assumptions?	After examining the facts, how has your experience of the event changed or remained the same?

What is the emotion that you want to change?	What event lead to you experiencing this emotion?	Are there any judgements or drastic statements in your description of this event?

What are your interpretations and assumptions about the facts?	What errors can you identify in your interpretations and assumptions?	After examining the facts, how has your experience of the event changed or remained the same?

What is the emotion that you want to change?	What event lead to you experiencing this emotion?	Are there any judgements or drastic statements in your description of this event?

What are your interpretations and assumptions about the facts?	What errors can you identify in your interpretations and assumptions?	After examining the facts, how has your experience of the event changed or remained the same?

What is the emotion that you want to change?	What event lead to you experiencing this emotion?	Are there any judgements or drastic statements in your description of this event?

What are your interpretations and assumptions about the facts?	What errors can you identify in your interpretations and assumptions?	After examining the facts, how has your experience of the event changed or remained the same?

Taking a closer look at self-criticism

The following activity can help you examine your self-criticism and help you identify steps that you can take to improve yourself in areas that you feel less confident.

Self-criticism Worksheet:

What are your self-critical statements?	How can you pursue progress rather than perfection?	How can you change your self-statements to support your progress?

What are your self-critical statements?	How can you pursue progress rather than perfection?	How can you change your self-statements to support your progress?

What are your self-critical statements?	How can you pursue progress rather than perfection?	How can you change your self-statements to support your progress?

Cultivating loving-kindness

Practicing loving-kindness can promote positive emotions and compassion towards ourselves and others. The practice of loving-kindness comes from Buddhist meditation and is about sending warm wishes to oneself and others. When beginning this practice, start by focusing on a loved one for the first several practices before offering this towards yourself. Throughout your loving kindness practice, keep your warm wishes sincere. The exercise below is a loving-kindness practice that you can utilize to begin incorporating this tool into your life. There are also many resources for loving kindness practices that you can find online.

Loving-kindness practice

Find yourself in a comfortable seated positive. Allowing your gaze to rest on a spot on the floor in front of you, take a few moments to check in with your body.

When you are ready, allow the eyes to close. Allow the breath to continue to deepen.

As you notice thoughts or distractions, simply acknowledge them without judgement before bringing your focus back to your breath.

Continue to focus on your breath.

Imagine the person that you intend to focus your loving kindness on today. Engage your senses to bring this person into your focus.

Select one or two warm wishes that you have for this person and continue to repeat these wishes slowly while feeling into the meaning of each word. Continue this until you feel completing surrounded by loving kindness. Warm wishes could include "may you feel safe and protected" or "may you be healthy in body and mind."

If you find your mind wandering, simply notice this before gently bringing your focus back to your breathe and warm wishes.

To end this practice, allow the eyes to slowly open and relax in front of you. Take your time to incorporate this practice before getting up and moving into the rest of your day.

Routines

Routines have shown to promote a sense of control and decrease distractions before and during sport performance. Routines can involve self-talk including both instructional and motivational self-talk. Routines can also involve meditation and relaxation skills.

What are your current routines prior to running?

What routines help to bring you into the present moment?

What can you do to improve your current routines to increase your concentration while running?

Mental imagery

Mental imagery is creating an experience in your mind using all of your senses. Imagery allows you to have an experience in a controlled and safe manner. Imagery has purpose and is used consciously. Imagery can be used to improve concentration as well as to improve performance, confidence, and relaxation. When using imagery, use vividness and focus on your success. For example, when utilizing imagery to improve concentration for running performance, imagine yourself utilizing your concentration perfectly to maintain your running form utilizing as much detail as possible. It is important to involve as many senses as possible into your imagery to promote vividness and knowing your learning style can further enhance your experience.

- Visual learning: Visual learners obtain information most effectively and prefer to learn through sight. During mental imagery, these learners can utilize additional visual cues to enhance their imagery.

- Experiential learning: Experiential learners learn best through doing. These learners can utilize the imagery of engaging in activities during their mental imagery to enhance this activity.

- Auditory learning: Auditory Learners prefer to obtain information through auditory cues. These learners can benefit from focusing on auditory senses during their imagery activities.

Internal versus external imagery

Internal imagery is being utilized when you imagine yourself doing something from your point of view while external imagery refers to seeing yourself in the third person during your imagery practice. Both can be useful and experimenting with both can help you determine which may be most beneficial for you.

6 ENERGY MANAGEMENT

This chapter will help you to manage your energy and implement relaxation skills to improve your training and performance. Take a few minutes to answer the following questions about your current energy management and relaxation skills:

How often do you consciously check in about how you are feeling during the day?

How often do you check in with your body?

Do you ask yourself "am I relaxed right now?" If so, how often?

How do you notice when you are not relaxed?

What do you do when you realize that you are worried, stressed, or anxious?

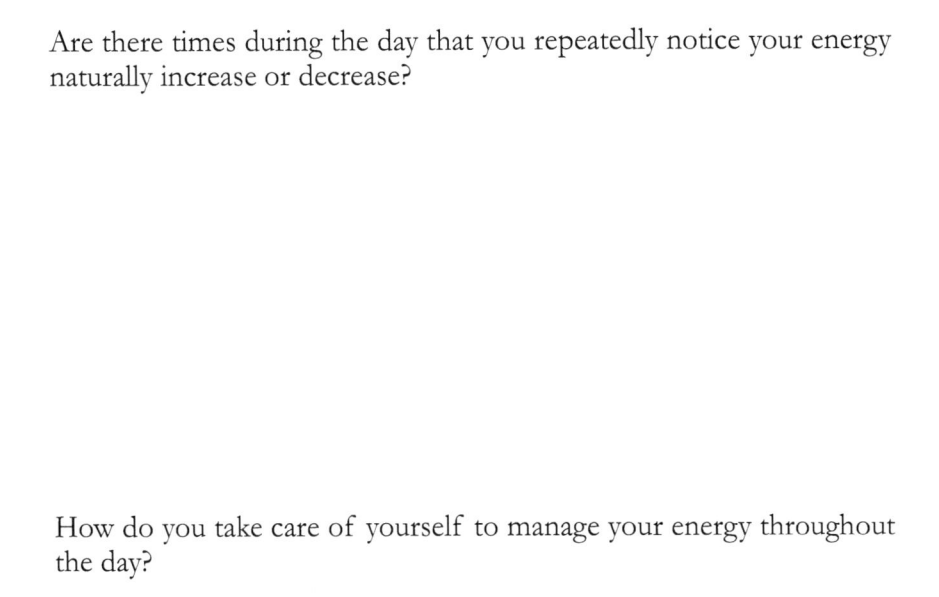

Are there times during the day that you repeatedly notice your energy naturally increase or decrease?

How do you take care of yourself to manage your energy throughout the day?

Coping skills

Coping skills are tools that we use to help us remain balanced and functioning well throughout the day. Coping skills can be different for everyone. People find certain techniques work better for them than others. Experiment with the different coping techniques mentioned in this chapter to see which may help you manage your energy and promote relaxation throughout your day. Note which skills help inspire you, relax you, and boost your energy. Please add to the following list with other skills that you utilize to manage your energy.

Coping Skills List:

- Sensory awareness check-in
- Body scan activity
- Progressive relaxation activity
- Deep breathing exercise
- Physical exercise
- Journal
- Draw or paint
- Sing
- Dance
- Bake
- Spend time with a pet
- Read a book
- Meditate
- Listen to music
- Take a shower or bath
- Pray
- Spend time outside
- Yoga
- Do a puzzle
- Listen to an inspiring podcast
- Spend time with others who inspire you
- Garden
- Learn something new
- Do something for someone else
- Talk with a friend
- Go for a walk
- Plan a trip
- Clean or reorganize your home
- Volunteer
- Make a gratitude list
- Use imagery
- Other:
- Other:
- Other:
- Other:
- Other:
- Other:
- Other:

Many of the skills in the coping skills list above are self-explanatory, but some benefit from further explanation. Some of these skills are explored in further detail below.

Deep breathing

Allow your breath to deepen. Place your hand on your low belly and notice your hand rising and falling with every breath. Count your breaths in order to help your mind focus on your relaxing deep breathing. Allow your breath to lengthen even more on the exhale to promote deeper relaxation.

Gratitude list

Develop a list of things that you are grateful for. Share this list with a friend or display it somewhere where you will see it regularly.

Sensory awareness check-in

This activity is about checking in with your senses. Find a comfortable position and use the following questions to help you.

1. Can you feel your chest and belly raising and lower with each breath?

2. Can you feel the weight of your body sinking into the floor?

3. Can you imagine sitting at the beach with the sun beating down on your skin?

4. Can you feel the air against her face?

5. Can you feel your arms relaxing?

6. Can you notice one leg containing more tension that the other leg?

7. Can you notice any smells?

8. Can you imagine the scent of fresh air after a rain?

9. Can you imagine floating on a cloud?

10. Can you notice your right toes and then your left toes?

11. Can you imaging looking at a beautiful landscape?

12. Can you imagine eating an orange? Engaging all your senses from feeling the sensations as you peel the skin away to expose the bright fruit within to smelling the citrus.

13. Can you feel one leg weighing heavier than the other leg?

14. Can you notice the sensations and tastes in your mouth?

Body scan

- Find a comfortable position either seated or laying down. Allow your gaze to softly rest on the floor in front of you.

- Bring your attention to your breath. Allow your eyes to close.

- Take several deep breaths and allow your body to relax.

- Bring your attention to the toes on your right foot. While continuing to pay attention to your breathing, notice to sensation in the toes of your right foot. Allow your mind to inquire what you are feeling in this part of your body. Continue to allow your attention to remain on the toes of your right foot for several minutes before moving to the arch and heel this foot.

- Inquire again about what you are feeling in this part of your body. Notice the weight of your foot on the floor.

- Next move up the body towards your right ankle. Bringing your attention to your right ankle, ask yourself what you are feeling in this part of your body. Notice any sensations on your skin. Spend several minutes focusing on your right ankle.

- Bring your attention to your calf. Notice any sensations and inquire what you are feeling in your right calf.

- Continue this inquiry as your bring your attention to your knee, then upper legs, and then follow the same process with the same body parts on your left side.

- Bring your attention your pelvis. Noticing the sensation of weight on the floor and inquiring what you are feeling in this part of your body.

- Continue this practice as you bring your attention to your lower back, then stomach, and then your chest. Continue to focus on these body parts one at a time while inquiring "what am I feeling?"

- Notice your breath. Notice the rising and falling of your belly as your breath moves like a wave in your body.

- Drawing your attention to your right hand, move your attention and inquiry up the right arm and into the shoulder.

- Repeat with your left hand, then arm, and then your shoulder.

- Finally bring your attention to your neck, then chin, then mouth, then tongue, then nose, then cheeks, then eyes, then forehead, and finally to the very top of your head.

- When thoughts or distractions arise during this body scan, simply notice them and gently bring your attention back to your body and your breath. Distractions are common during this activity. Please respond to them with compassion.

- Once you have moved through your entire body, take several deep breaths as your body continues to relax.

- When you are ready, you may open your eyes and allow your gaze to rest softly on the floor in front of you.

- Take another few breaths here before completing this body scan and moving into the rest of your day.

Progressive relaxation

Progressive relaxation is a technique involving tensing and relaxing different muscles in a systematic way. This type of relaxation can promote both physical and mental relaxation.

- Find a comfortable position either seated or laying down. Allow your gaze to softly rest on the floor in front of you.

- Bring your attention to your breath. Allow your eyes to close.

- Take several deep breaths and allow your body to relax.

- Similar to the body scan, bring your attention to each part of your body one at a time beginning with your right foot and working up to the top of your head.

- As you bring focus to each body part, first tense and then relax each muscle one at a time. When tensing your muscles, hold the tension for a count of five. When relaxing your muscles, really allow the tension to drift away.

- When thoughts or distractions arise during this progressive relaxation, simply notice them and gently bring your attention back to your body and your breath. Distractions are common and it is best to respond to them with compassion.

- Once you have moved through your entire body, take several deep breaths as your body continues to relax.

- When you are ready, you may open your eyes and allow your gaze to rest softly on the floor in front of you.

- Take another few breaths here before completing this progressive relaxation and moving into the rest of your day.

Coping ahead

Coping skills are excellent to use the moment when you discover that you are out of balance. Coping ahead is another way to use coping skills. This technique involves implementing coping skills before getting out of balance. This may be especially useful when anticipating a challenging activity. Coping ahead may be especially effective in managing anxiety before a race. Part of coping ahead also involves caring for the body including maintaining proper nutrition, obtaining sleep, and spending time getting exercise.

7 CARING FOR THE BODY

Runners care for their bodies in a variety of different ways. Caring for the body can reduce the risk of injuries as well as the risk of burn out. Nutrition, sleep, and rest are critical for recovery and will be discussed first in this chapter. Other common recovery techniques, including baths, compression gear, sensory deprivation tanks, and massage/bodywork, will be addressed only briefly in this chapter. Finally, this chapter will present information about yoga for runners and will include two yoga routines to incorporate into your training if you so desire. Runners claim that the approaches mentioned in this chapter help them to perform better. Every body is different. Do your research and experiment with what works best for you.

Basic nutrition

Practicing good overall nutrition can provide a lot of support to your running. After your run, refueling with carbohydrates and protein is very important. Try to consume this within the 30 minutes following your workout. Fluids are also very important before, during, and after a run. For long runs, it is recommended to drink 16 oz fluid beforehand & approximately 8 oz every 20 minutes during the run. When preparing for a long run, drink fluids and eat carbohydrates and protein approximately 2 hours before your run.

Sleep

Sleep is important for everybody and especially for runners. Common techniques to improve sleep include the following:

- Limiting naps during the day

- Exercising regularly during the day but not right before sleep

- Avoiding caffeine and tobacco before bedtime as well as steering clear of food that is heavy, rich, or spicy or foods that can trigger indigestion before sleep

- Getting natural light exposure during the day

- Limiting screen time before bed

- Engaging in relaxation activities before bed such as taking a bath or using essential oils

- Establishing bedtime routines to cue your body that you will be going to sleep soon

- When having trouble going to sleep, instead of laying in bed for a long time, get up and do relaxing activities such as reading a book or stretching but do not utilize bright lights or engage in activities that include screen time

Rest

Rest is also vital for runners to excel and to mitigate injuries. Every training plan should include rest days and easy runs. It is important not to skip these rest days and to appreciate easy runs as part of recovery. Many runners use additional techniques to aid in recovery. Common recovery techniques include the following:

Baths

Ice baths are a common recovery activity for runners because they are known to decrease tissue breakdown and inflammation. The duration of these baths should be kept short. Epsom salt baths are another popular recovery tool. The heat and Epsom salt promote muscle relaxation. The general rule of thumb is to spend 20-30 minutes in the bath when using Epsom salts.

Compression

While compression gear claims to increase circulation and decrease blood lactate concentration, some runners wear compression gear during runs because they feel it provides them with additional support. Calf sleeves and compression socks tend to be especially prevalent in the running community.

Sensory deprivation tanks

Deprivation tanks utilize high levels of Epsom salt to allow the user to float. The tank is dark and silent to deprive the user of sensory input, and the water is maintained to remain at body temperature. In addition to physical benefits, users have reported mental benefits including increased relaxation.

Massage/ bodywork

Massage and other bodywork including Rolfing and Hellerwork can benefit runners by increasing muscle relaxation as well as aiding in posture and form. Rolfing and Hellerwork bodywork examine muscle structure to address asymmetries, and any type of massage can help reduce tension and restore optimal range of motion.

Yoga routines

While some runners experience a benefit from keeping their

muscles tighter, many claim that yoga and stretching support their running. Yoga can support runners to address their asymmetries and to tune in with their bodies. Moreover, the breath in yoga aids focus and can be used to ease tension in the body and mind.

The following yoga routines have been designed to support runners physically and mentally. Feel free to experiment with adding these routines to your training routine to see how they may benefit you.

Sequence for runners #1

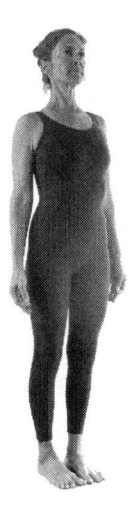

•**Mountain pose:** Begin by standing with your feet parallel and shoulder distance apart. Notice strength and stability as you engage your leg muscles and core muscles. Allow the arms to rest alongside your body with your palms facing forward. Draw the shoulder blades down and back to support on opening in your chest. Notice your breathing. Remain in this pose for 10-20 breaths.

Benefits: Mountain pose is the foundation for all the other yoga postures. It aligns the entire body, stretches the legs, and steadies the mind and the breath.

•**Forward fold:** From mountain pose, with your inhale reach your arms to the sky and, with your knees slightly bent, exhale fold forward from your hip joints and allow your upper body to extend towards the ground. Allow your arms to relax as they lengthen towards your toes. Feel the strength in your legs as you continue to activate these muscles. Remain in this pose for 5-10 breaths.

Benefits: Forward fold stretches the entire back side of the body, primarily stretching the backs of the legs and lengthening the spine.

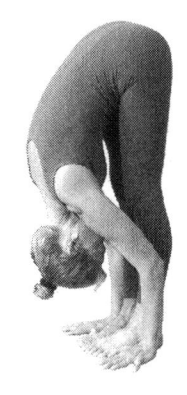

- **Downward facing dog pose:** Starting on the floor on your hands and knees, spread your palms and tuck your toes. With your inhale draw your shoulder blades back towards your waist and with your exhale bring your knees up away from the floor. Allow the legs to straighten or maintain a slight bend in the knees. Draw your sitting bones towards the sky as you feel your torso and arms lengthening. Continue to keep your arms and core muscles activated as you push and extend from your hands. Remain in this pose for 5-10 breaths or as long as you feel comfortable. To exit this post, follow your exhale by bending your knees to the floor. *This pose can be modified by placing the hands on the wall or on a chair.

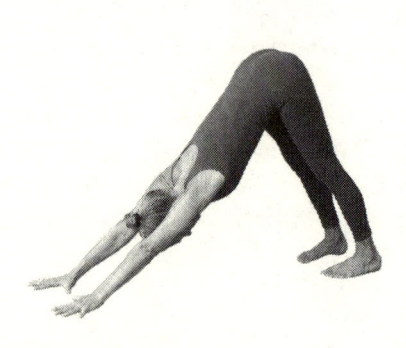

Benefits: Downward facing dog pose is one of the best poses for runners as a warm up and post running stretch. As it strengthens the upper body, primarily wrists, arms and shoulders, it also opens the chest and elongates the spine, so one's breathing is improved. This pose also stretches the entire back body, primarily the hamstrings, calf muscles and achilles tendons.

- **Plank pose:** From downward-facing dog pose, allow your exhale to lead as you draw your torso forward until your shoulders are directly above your wrists. Continue to activate your leg and core muscles. Bring your attention to your shoulder blades drawing down the back and broadening away from the spine. While maintaining a straight line from heels to shoulders, feel a lifting in your thighs towards the sky and maintain your core muscles to maintain support in this pose. Remain in this position for 5-10 breaths or as long as you feel comfortable. To exit this pose, simply bend the knees to rest the knees on the floor.

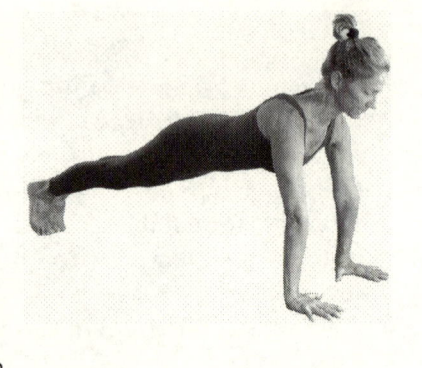

Benefits: Plank pose strengthens the upper body primarily the arms, wrists, shoulders as well as the core torso muscles.

- **Cobra pose:** Starting by laying flat on the floor with your stomach resting on the ground, place your hands on the floor under your shoulders. Spread the fingers and allow the elbows to remain close to the body. With your next inhale, lift your chest away from the floor as you extend your arms. Feel the length throughout your body from your toes up your back and into the top of your head. Continue to draw the shoulder blades down and into the back. Lift the chest upwards only to where you feel comfortable and maintain comfortable breathing throughout this pose. Remain in this pose for 5-10 breaths before lengthening your spine as you exhale the chest back to the floor.

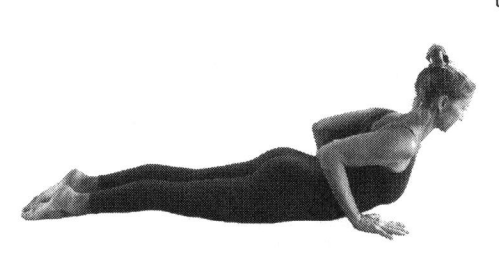

Benefits: Cobra strengthens the upper back and spinal extensor muscles which helps with overall improved posture alignment and breathing.

- **Extended side angle pose:** Return to mountain pose. With your exhale, step your feet about 3.5-4 feet apart. Rotate your right foot and leg 90 degrees to your right. With your next inhale, draw your arms up and parallel to the floor. Allow your right knee to bend so that your right leg forms a 90 degree angle with the knee in line above the ankle. With your next exhale, allow your upper body to extend and hinge from your hip to the right as you bring your right arm down alongside your right foot. You may choose to rest your right hand on a block or allow the elbow to sit on the thigh of your right leg instead of having the right hand rest on the floor depending on your flexibility. Pressing your left foot into the ground, bring your left arm alongside your left ear and allow your gaze to turn towards your left upper arm. Feel the strength in your core as you lengthen toward the top of your head in this pose.

Remain in this pose for 5-10 breaths. To exit this pose, with your inhale draw your left arm towards that sky as you draw your upper body into a vertical position and straighten the right leg while maintaining the alignment of your front knee. Return the right foot and leg to a forward facing position before repeating this pose on the left side.

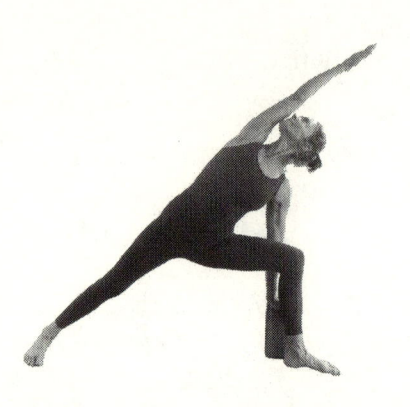

Benefits: Side angle pose stretches and strengthens the feet, arches, ankles and knees. It also opens the adductors and hamstrings as well as strengthens the quadriceps and abductors of the hips, elongates the spine and opens the chest.

- **Triangle pose:** Beginning in Mountain pose, exhale your feet apart about 3.5-4 feet. With your next inhale lift your arms to stretch on either side of you parallel to the floor. Rotate your right foot 90 degrees and allow the left foot to rotate slightly. Allow your right leg to rotate to the right while keeping muscles activated. With your next inhale lengthen your spine towards the the sky and with your next exhale hinge from the hip to the right side. Allow your right arm to reach towards the floor or to rest on the shin of your right leg as you reach your right arm up towards the sky. Finally, allow your torso, chest, and gaze to turn skyward towards your left hand. Remain in this pose for 5-10 breaths. To exit this pose, follow your inhale as you push from your heel and reach through your left hand to bring your torso back to a vertical position. Straightening your leg and rotating it back to the front of the mat before repeating this pose on the left side.

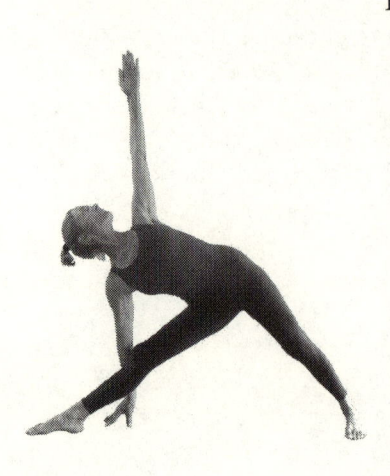

Benefits: Triangle pose stretches and strengthens the feet, arches, ankles and knees. It also opens the adductors and hamstrings as well as strengthens the quadriceps and abductor muscles of the hips, elongates the spine and opens the chest.

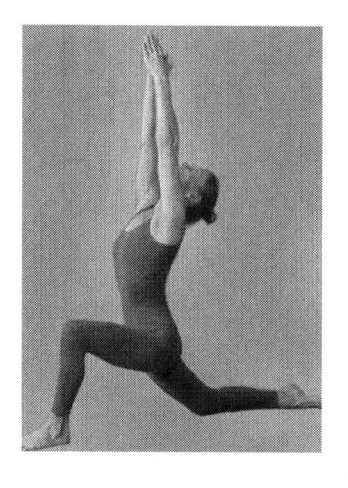

- **Lunge:** Beginning in downward facing dog pose, draw the right knee into the chest with your inhale and place the right foot on the floor in front of you. Allow the left foot to slide towards the back of the mat and the left knee to rest onto the floor. Draw the spine up and place your hands on your right knee. Check to make sure that your right knee is at a 90 degree angle with the knee in line with the ankle. As you experience this stretch in your lower body, feel the upper body lengthening with the top of the head reaching towards the sky. Follow the breath and remain in this pose to 5-10 breaths or as long as you feel comfortable. Repeat this stretch on the other side.

Benefits: Lunges are great stretches for the hip flexor muscles including the quadriceps, psoas muscles and inner groin. Additionally, as the front body is stretched, the back body including the spinal extensor muscles are strengthened.

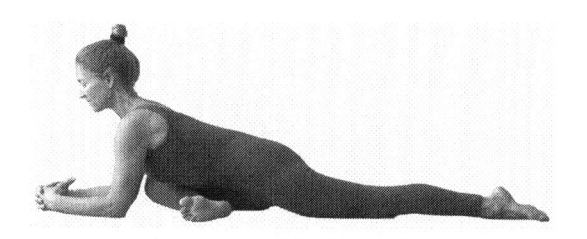

- **Pigeon pose:** Beginning with your knees in line with your hips on all fours, bring your right knee forward on the floor in front of you and turn your right shin under your torso with your right foot in front of your left foot. Allow the left leg to lengthen back as the left knee straightens. Bring your torso closer to the floor as you extend your arms in front of you. Lower your upper body as low as you feel comfortable maintaining an easy breath. Remain in this pose for 5-10 breaths or as long as you feel comfortable.

Benefits: Pigeon pose stretches the abductor muscles and generally increases mobility of the hips.

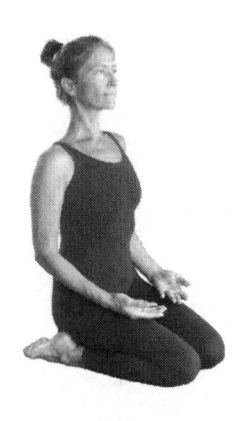

•**Hero pose:** Beginning by kneeling on the floor, touch your inner knees together while sliding your feet apart. Find your feet slightly wider than your hips. On your exhale slowly sit down between your feet. If this is uncomfortable, place a block or blanket under your hips to reduce the intensity of this stretch. While feeling a stretch in your lower body, allow the top of your head to extend towards the sky. Feel the lengthening in your upper body and ease in your breath. Remain in this pose for 10-20 breaths or as long as you feel comfortable.

Benefits: Hero pose increases flexibility to the ankles, arches, and feet as well as to the quadricep muscles.

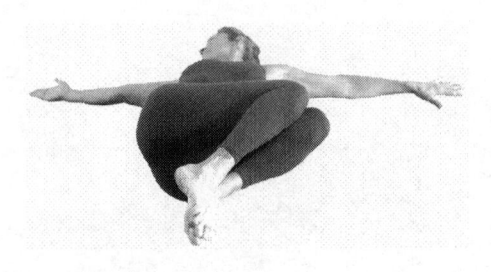

- **Reclining twist:** Beginning by laying down with the back supported on the floor. Bend the knees so that the bottom of the feet are resting on the floor. Extend both arms out to the sides of your body. With your inhale bring the legs up and with your next exhale move the legs to the left to allow the legs to lower to the floor. With your next inhale feel the spine lengthen up towards the top of your head and turn your gaze towards your right hand which continues to extend out from your shoulder along the floor next to you. Remain in this pose for 5-10 breaths or as long as you feel comfortable. To exit this pose, inhale the legs up before repeating this pose on the other side for symmetry.

Benefits: Reclining twists utilize gravity to facilitate stretching and releasing tension out of the body. Specifically, twists stretch muscles of the hips, rib cage and shoulders while toning the abdominal muscles and revitalizing the spine.

- **Corpse pose:** This pose can be done on a yoga mat and or on a blanket for additional support. Make sure that your body is supported equally and remains a comfortable temperature. Lay down with your back resting into the floor. Close the eyes and rest the arms alongside our torso with palms facing upwards. Allow the breath to guide the body is it relaxes into the support of the floor. This is an important pose to integrate your practice and transition from your yoga practice to the rest of your day. Remain in this pose for 5+ minutes.

Benefits: Corpse is an important posture to relax and renew the entire body. It is calming for the nervous system and helps bring overall balance to the body and mind.

Sequence for runners #2

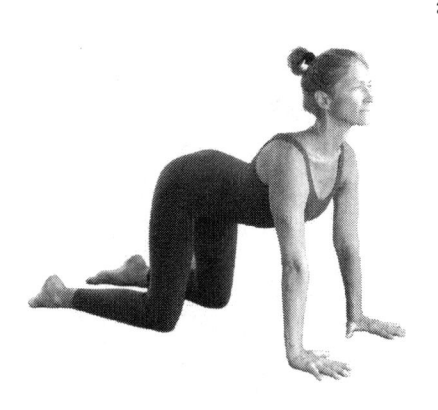

- **Cat/cow:** Beginning on hands and knees with the back flat and parallel to the floor, align your knees to be directly below your hips and your wrists and elbows directly below your shoulders. With your next inhale allow your spine to extend and your hips and chest to move towards the sky and draw the shoulder blades down the back. On your next exhale allow your spine to flex and round towards the sky drawing in the belly. On your next inhale allow your hips and chest to move towards the sky again and on your next exhale allowing the spine to round towards the sky again. Follow your breath to repeat these motions as many times as you desire.

Benefits: Cat/cow primarily stretches and strengthens the muscles along the back and front of the spine as well as mobilizes the pelvis, spine, rib cage, and shoulder blades.

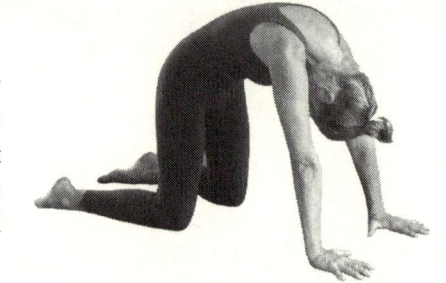

- **Mountain pose:** Begin by standing with your feet parallel and shoulder distance apart. Notice strength and stability as you engage your leg muscles and core muscles . Allow the arms to rest alongside your body with your palms facing forward. Draw the shoulder blades down and back to support on opening in your chest. Notice your breathing. Remain in this pose for 10-20 breaths.

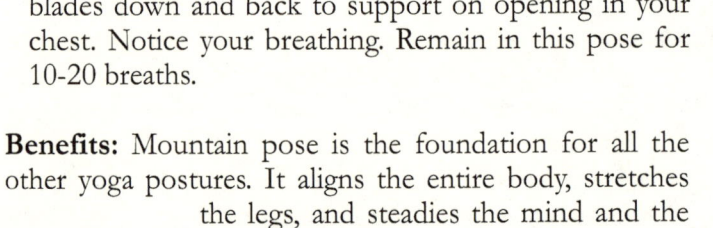

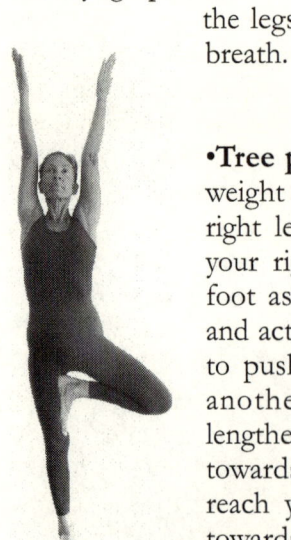

Benefits: Mountain pose is the foundation for all the other yoga postures. It aligns the entire body, stretches the legs, and steadies the mind and the breath.

•**Tree pose:** Beginning in Mountain pose, shift your weight on to your left side and begin to draw the right leg up as you reach your right hand to meet your right foot. Using your hand, place your right foot as high up on your left side as is comfortable and activate the muscles in your right leg and left leg to push the right foot and the left thigh into one another. From this tension, feel the spine lengthening and the top of the head reaching towards the sky. Place your hands on your hips or reach your arms parallel to one another and up towards the sky. Allow your gaze to rest out in front of you on the floor. Allow the chest to open in this pose and feel yourself grounded through your left foot on the floor. Remain in this pose for 5-10 breaths before releasing the right leg to return to mountain pose on the exhalation. Repeat this pose on the other side. *Maintaining a fixed gaze on the floor about 4-5 feet in front of you can help your balance in this pose. If you lose balance at any point during this pose, simply regain your balance before stepping back into this pose. This pose can also be modified by standing against a wall or near a wall to assist with balance.

Benefits: Tree pose strengthens the external rotators and opens the adductors and quadriceps of the hips, elongates the spine, opens the chest, and steadies the mind.

- **Downward facing dog pose:** Starting on the floor on your hands and knees, spread your palms and tuck your toes. With your inhale draw your shoulder blades back towards your waist and with your exhale bring your knees up away from the floor. Allow the legs to straighten or maintain a slight bend in the knees. Draw your sitting bones towards the sky as you feel your torso and arms lengthening. Continue to keep your arms and core muscles activated as you push and extend from your hands. Remain in this pose for 5-10 breaths or as long as you feel comfortable. To exit this post, follow your exhale by bending your knees to the floor. *This pose can be modified by placing the hands on the wall or on a chair.

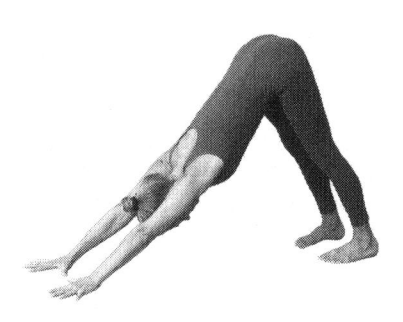

Benefits: Downward facing dog pose is one of the best poses for runners as a warm up and post running stretch. As it strengthens the upper body, primarily wrists, arms and shoulders, it also opens the chest and elongates the spine, so one's breathing is improved. This pose also stretches the entire back body, primarily the hamstrings, calf muscles and achilles tendons.

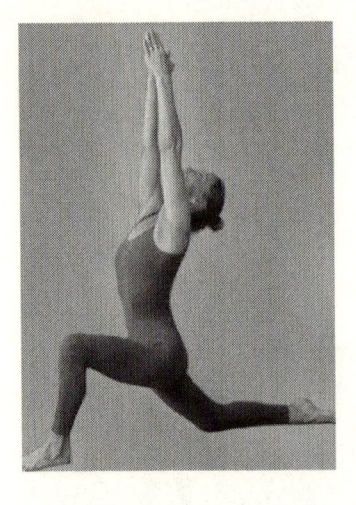

•**Lunge:** Beginning in downward facing dog pose, draw the right knee into the chest with your inhale and place the right foot on the floor in front of you. Allow the left foot to slide towards the back of the mat and the left knee to rest onto the floor. Draw the spine up and place your hands on your right knee. Check to make sure that your right knee is at a 90 degree angle with the knee in line with the ankle. As you experience this stretch in your lower body, feel the upper body lengthening with the top of the head reaching towards the sky. Follow the breath and remain in this pose to 5-10 breaths or as long as you feel comfortable. Repeat this stretch on the other side.

Benefits: Lunges are great stretches for the hip flexor muscles including the quadriceps, psoas muscles and inner groin. Additionally, as the front body is stretched, the back body including the spinal extensor muscles are strengthened.

• **Head to knee pose:** Begin by sitting upright on the floor with the legs straight out in front of you. Inhale as you extend the spine reaching the top of the head towards the sky and fold the right leg with the heal as close to the pelvis as you feel comfortable and the knee resting towards the floor on your right side. With your next exhale lengthening the spine forward and allowing the arms to extend towards your left foot. Continue to lengthen and feel supported by the breath in this stretch. Maintain ease in your breath and remain in this pose for 10-20 breaths or as long as you feel comfortable. To exit this pose, follow your inhalation as you lengthen the spine up into an upright seated position and release the leg before repeating this pose on the other side.

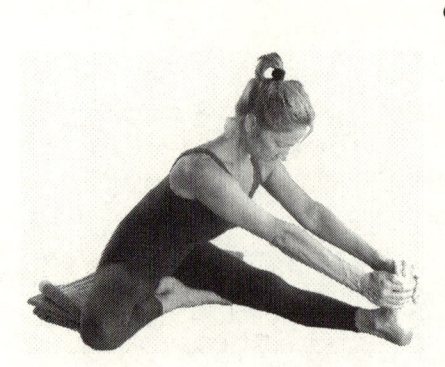

Benefits: Head to knee pose is a calming pose that primarily stretches the hamstrings of the extended leg and the adductors of the bent leg while elongating the spine.

- **Bound angle pose:** Beginning with your legs straight out in front of you in a seated position, with your exhale bend your knees so that your heels are drawn as close to your pelvis as you feel comfortable and your knees are resting towards the floor on either side of you. With your next inhale lengthen the upper body towards the sky and then fold forward from the hip joints as far as you feel comfortable. Remain in this pose for 10-20 breaths or as long as you feel comfortable. To exit this pose, inhale the upper body towards the sky before releasing the legs to extend out in front of you.

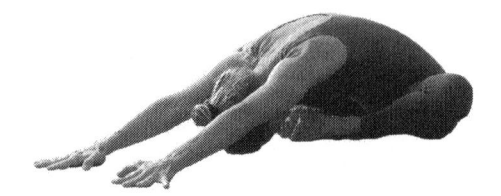

Benefits: Bound angle pose is great for the health of the pelvic area. Specifically, it stretches the adductor muscles and quadriceps and generally increases the mobility of the hips.

- **Hero pose:** Beginning by kneeling on the floor, touch your inner knees together while sliding your feet apart. Find your feet slightly wider than your hips. On your exhale slowly sit down between your feet. If this is uncomfortable, place a block or blanket under your hips to reduce the intensity of this stretch. While feeling a stretch in your lower body, allow the top of your head to extend towards the sky. Feel the lengthening in your upper body and ease in your breath. Remain in this pose for 10-20 breaths or as long as you feel comfortable.

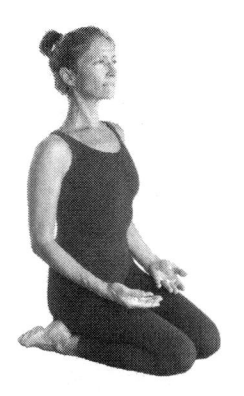

Benefits: Hero pose increases flexibility to the ankles, arches, and feet as well as to the quadricep muscles.

- **Cows face:** Begin by sitting with the legs extended in front of you and the spine in a vertical position. Bending your knees with your feet on the floor, place your left foot under your right knee and placing the right knee on top of the left. Place the right foot on the outside of your left hip so that both heels are located on either side of your hips and your sitting bones remain on the floor. With your next inhale extend the spine reaching the top of the head towards the sky and with your next exhale allow the upper body to fold forward at the hip joints. Continue to lengthen the spine forward as much as your feel comfortable without straining the back.

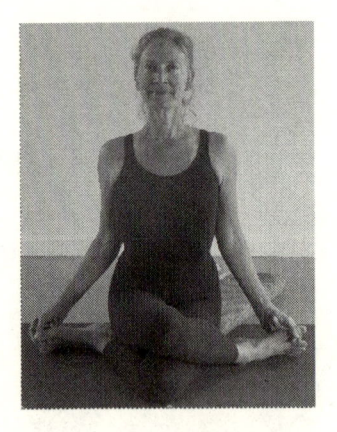

Benefits: Cows face pose for the lower body stretches the spine and the abductor muscles of the hips and strengthens the ankles.

- **Child's pose:** Beginning by kneeling on the floor with your feet touching, sit back onto your heels. With your next exhale extend your spine as you fold forward to rest your upper body onto your thighs. Allow your arms to rest on the floor alongside your torso. Allow your forehead to be supported by the floor. Follow your breath as your muscles relax and sink into the floor. Remain in this pose for 20+ breaths or as long as you feel comfortable.

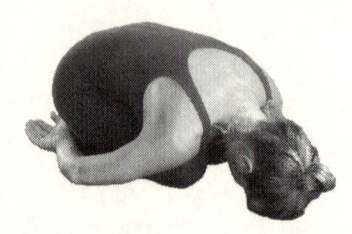

Benefits: Child's pose helps release tension and offers a gentle warm up for the entire spine, particularly the lower back. It also stretches the fronts of the ankles and quadriceps of the thighs.

- **Legs up the wall:** For this restorative pose, position yourself laying on your side with your sitting bones against a wall. When you're ready, swing your legs up the wall as you roll onto your back. Straighten the legs and allow them to feel supported by the wall. Relax your upper body as it sinks into the floor. Allow your arms to lay on either side of you next to your torso with palms facing up. You can do this pose on yoga mat and/or on a blanket for more support. Make sure that you are warm enough during this restorative pose. Slide yourself closer or farther away from the wall based on comfort. Remain in this pose for 2+ minutes or as long as you feel comfortable. This pose is considered an inversion pose and should be avoided during menstruation.

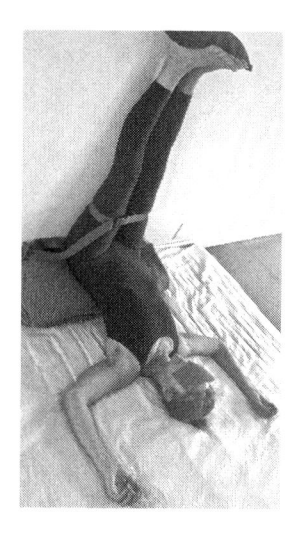

Benefits: Legs up the wall is a relaxing pose to calm the nervous system and the mind. It also gently elongates and stretches the backs of the legs.

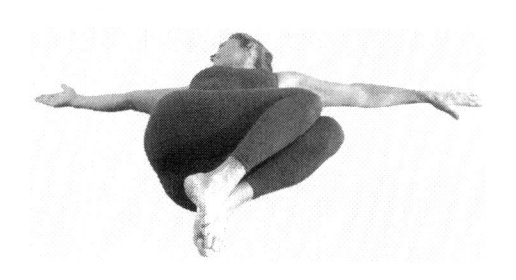

- **Reclining twist:** Beginning by laying down with the back supported on the floor. Bend the knees so that the bottom of the feet are resting on the floor. Extend both arms out to the sides of your body. With your inhale bring the legs up and with your next exhale move the legs to the left to allow the legs to lower to the floor. With your next inhale feel the spine lengthen up towards the top of your head and turn your gaze towards your right hand which continues to extend out from your shoulder along the floor next to you. Remain in this pose for 5-10 breaths or as long as you feel comfortable. To exit this pose, inhale the legs up before repeating this pose on the other side for symmetry.

Benefits: Reclining twists utilize gravity to facilitate stretching and releasing tension out of the body. Specifically, twists stretch muscles of the hips, rib cage and shoulders while toning the abdominal muscles and revitalizing the spine.

- **Corpse pose:** This pose can be done on a yoga mat and or on a blanket for additional support. Make sure that your body is supported equally and remains a comfortable temperature. Lay down with your back resting into the floor. Close the eyes and rest the arms alongside our torso with palms facing upwards. Allow the breath to guide the body is it relaxes into the support of the floor. This is an important pose to integrate your practice and transition from your yoga practice to the rest of your day. Remain in this pose for 5+ minutes.

Benefits: Corpse is an important posture to relax and renew the entire body. It is calming for the nervous system and helps bring overall balance to the body and mind.

8 TRAINING JOURNAL

This training journal is designed to support you in integrating the information that you have obtained throughout this workbook into your training. Please use this journal in whatever way you feel would benefit you most.

Date:

My training goals for this week are:

I can mitigate obstacles this week by:

Day of the week	Distance/Speed	What was the purpose of this specific run?	How did I feel before, during, and after this run?
Monday			
Tuesday			
Wednesday			
Thursday			

Day of the week	Distance/Speed	What was the purpose of this specific run?	How did I feel before, during, and after this run?
Friday			
Saturday			
Sunday			

This week, I am most proud of myself for:

Date:

My training goals for this week are:

I can mitigate obstacles this week by:

Day of the week	Distance/Speed	What was the purpose of this specific run?	How did I feel before, during, and after this run?
Monday			
Tuesday			
Wednesday			
Thursday			

Day of the week	Distance/Speed	What was the purpose of this specific run?	How did I feel before, during, and after this run?
Friday			
Saturday			
Sunday			

This week, I am most proud of myself for:

Date:

My training goals for this week are:

I can mitigate obstacles this week by:

Day of the week	Distance/Speed	What was the purpose of this specific run?	How did I feel before, during, and after this run?
Monday			
Tuesday			
Wednesday			
Thursday			

Day of the week	Distance/Speed	What was the purpose of this specific run?	How did I feel before, during, and after this run?
Friday			
Saturday			
Sunday			

This week, I am most proud of myself for:

Date:

My training goals for this week are:

I can mitigate obstacles this week by:

Day of the week	Distance/Speed	What was the purpose of this specific run?	How did I feel before, during, and after this run?
Monday			
Tuesday			
Wednesday			
Thursday			

Day of the week	Distance/Speed	What was the purpose of this specific run?	How did I feel before, during, and after this run?
Friday			
Saturday			
Sunday			

Obstacles will arise. It's how we respond to those obstacles that matters most. Take a moment to check in regarding how you are handling obstacles. Is there room for improvement? How so?

Date:

My training goals for this week are:

I can mitigate obstacles this week by:

Day of the week	Distance/Speed	What was the purpose of this specific run?	How did I feel before, during, and after this run?
Monday			
Tuesday			
Wednesday			
Thursday			

Day of the week	Distance/Speed	What was the purpose of this specific run?	How did I feel before, during, and after this run?
Friday			
Saturday			
Sunday			

This week, I am most proud of myself for:

Date:

My training goals for this week are:

I can mitigate obstacles this week by:

Day of the week	Distance/Speed	What was the purpose of this specific run?	How did I feel before, during, and after this run?
Monday			
Tuesday			
Wednesday			
Thursday			

Day of the week	Distance/Speed	What was the purpose of this specific run?	How did I feel before, during, and after this run?
Friday			
Saturday			
Sunday			

This week, I am most proud of myself for:

Date:

My training goals for this week are:

I can mitigate obstacles this week by:

Day of the week	Distance/Speed	What was the purpose of this specific run?	How did I feel before, during, and after this run?
Monday			
Tuesday			
Wednesday			
Thursday			

Day of the week	Distance/Speed	What was the purpose of this specific run?	How did I feel before, during, and after this run?
Friday			
Saturday			
Sunday			

Track your successes. Take a moment to reflect on your successes during this training cycle so far. What has helped you to achieve these successes? What can you do to promote continued success?

Date:

My training goals for this week are:

I can mitigate obstacles this week by:

Day of the week	Distance/Speed	What was the purpose of this specific run?	How did I feel before, during, and after this run?
Monday			
Tuesday			
Wednesday			
Thursday			

Day of the week	Distance/Speed	What was the purpose of this specific run?	How did I feel before, during, and after this run?
Friday			
Saturday			
Sunday			

This week, I am most proud of myself for:

Date:

My training goals for this week are:

I can mitigate obstacles this week by:

Day of the week	Distance/Speed	What was the purpose of this specific run?	How did I feel before, during, and after this run?
Monday			
Tuesday			
Wednesday			
Thursday			

Day of the week	Distance/Speed	What was the purpose of this specific run?	How did I feel before, during, and after this run?
Friday			
Saturday			
Sunday			

This week, I am most proud of myself for:

Date:

My training goals for this week are:

I can mitigate obstacles this week by:

Day of the week	Distance/Speed	What was the purpose of this specific run?	How did I feel before, during, and after this run?
Monday			
Tuesday			
Wednesday			
Thursday			

Day of the week	Distance/Speed	What was the purpose of this specific run?	How did I feel before, during, and after this run?
Friday			
Saturday			
Sunday			

This week, I am most proud of myself for:

Date:

My training goals for this week are:

I can mitigate obstacles this week by:

Day of the week	Distance/Speed	What was the purpose of this specific run?	How did I feel before, during, and after this run?
Monday			
Tuesday			
Wednesday			
Thursday			

Day of the week	Distance/Speed	What was the purpose of this specific run?	How did I feel before, during, and after this run?
Friday			
Saturday			
Sunday			

Take a moment to check in on your motivation and your goals. Are your goals challenging you? Are they attainable?

Date:

My training goals for this week are:

I can mitigate obstacles this week by:

Day of the week	Distance/Speed	What was the purpose of this specific run?	How did I feel before, during, and after this run?
Monday			
Tuesday			
Wednesday			
Thursday			

Day of the week	Distance/Speed	What was the purpose of this specific run?	How did I feel before, during, and after this run?
Friday			
Saturday			
Sunday			

This week, I am most proud of myself for:

Date:

My training goals for this week are:

I can mitigate obstacles this week by:

Day of the week	Distance/Speed	What was the purpose of this specific run?	How did I feel before, during, and after this run?
Monday			
Tuesday			
Wednesday			
Thursday			

Day of the week	Distance/Speed	What was the purpose of this specific run?	How did I feel before, during, and after this run?
Friday			
Saturday			
Sunday			

This week, I am most proud of myself for:

Date:

My training goals for this week are:

I can mitigate obstacles this week by:

Day of the week	Distance/Speed	What was the purpose of this specific run?	How did I feel before, during, and after this run?
Monday			
Tuesday			
Wednesday			
Thursday			

Day of the week	Distance/Speed	What was the purpose of this specific run?	How did I feel before, during, and after this run?
Friday			
Saturday			
Sunday			

This week, I am most proud of myself for:

Date:

My training goals for this week are:

I can mitigate obstacles this week by:

Day of the week	Distance/Speed	What was the purpose of this specific run?	How did I feel before, during, and after this run?
Monday			
Tuesday			
Wednesday			
Thursday			

Day of the week	Distance/Speed	What was the purpose of this specific run?	How did I feel before, during, and after this run?
Friday			
Saturday			
Sunday			

How are you progressing towards your goals? Take a moment to reflect on your training and on how it measures up to your specific goals. Are you on track? If not, what can you do to get back on track? Do your goals need to be adjusted?

Date:

My training goals for this week are:

I can mitigate obstacles this week by:

Day of the week	Distance/Speed	What was the purpose of this specific run?	How did I feel before, during, and after this run?
Monday			
Tuesday			
Wednesday			
Thursday			

Day of the week	Distance/Speed	What was the purpose of this specific run?	How did I feel before, during, and after this run?
Friday			
Saturday			
Sunday			

This week, I am most proud of myself for:

Date:

My training goals for this week are:

I can mitigate obstacles this week by:

Day of the week	Distance/Speed	What was the purpose of this specific run?	How did I feel before, during, and after this run?
Monday			
Tuesday			
Wednesday			
Thursday			

Day of the week	Distance/Speed	What was the purpose of this specific run?	How did I feel before, during, and after this run?
Friday			
Saturday			
Sunday			

This week, I am most proud of myself for:

Date:

My training goals for this week are:

I can mitigate obstacles this week by:

Day of the week	Distance/Speed	What was the purpose of this specific run?	How did I feel before, during, and after this run?
Monday			
Tuesday			
Wednesday			
Thursday			

Day of the week	Distance/Speed	What was the purpose of this specific run?	How did I feel before, during, and after this run?
Friday			
Saturday			
Sunday			

Take a moment to check in on how you are doing with sleep. A lack of sleep can contribute to challenges during your training cycle. If you feel that you are not getting enough sleep, how can you implement some changes to improve your sleep?

Date:

My training goals for this week are:

I can mitigate obstacles this week by:

Day of the week	Distance/Speed	What was the purpose of this specific run?	How did I feel before, during, and after this run?
Monday			
Tuesday			
Wednesday			
Thursday			

Day of the week	Distance/Speed	What was the purpose of this specific run?	How did I feel before, during, and after this run?
Friday			
Saturday			
Sunday			

This week, I am most proud of myself for:

Date:

My training goals for this week are:

I can mitigate obstacles this week by:

Day of the week	Distance/Speed	What was the purpose of this specific run?	How did I feel before, during, and after this run?
Monday			
Tuesday			
Wednesday			
Thursday			

Day of the week	Distance/Speed	What was the purpose of this specific run?	How did I feel before, during, and after this run?
Friday			
Saturday			
Sunday			

This week, I am most proud of myself for:

Date:

My training goals for this week are:

I can mitigate obstacles this week by:

Day of the week	Distance/Speed	What was the purpose of this specific run?	How did I feel before, during, and after this run?
Monday			
Tuesday			
Wednesday			
Thursday			

Day of the week	Distance/Speed	What was the purpose of this specific run?	How did I feel before, during, and after this run?
Friday			
Saturday			
Sunday			

How is your motivation at this point in your training cycle? Is it time to revisit your goals to remind yourself of what you're working towards?

Date:

My training goals for this week are:

I can mitigate obstacles this week by:

Day of the week	Distance/Speed	What was the purpose of this specific run?	How did I feel before, during, and after this run?
Monday			
Tuesday			
Wednesday			
Thursday			

Day of the week	Distance/Speed	What was the purpose of this specific run?	How did I feel before, during, and after this run?
Friday			
Saturday			
Sunday			

This week, I am most proud of myself for:

Date:

My training goals for this week are:

I can mitigate obstacles this week by:

Day of the week	Distance/Speed	What was the purpose of this specific run?	How did I feel before, during, and after this run?
Monday			
Tuesday			
Wednesday			
Thursday			

Day of the week	Distance/Speed	What was the purpose of this specific run?	How did I feel before, during, and after this run?
Friday			
Saturday			
Sunday			

This week, I am most proud of myself for:

Date:

My training goals for this week are:

I can mitigate obstacles this week by:

Day of the week	Distance/Speed	What was the purpose of this specific run?	How did I feel before, during, and after this run?
Monday			
Tuesday			
Wednesday			
Thursday			

Day of the week	Distance/Speed	What was the purpose of this specific run?	How did I feel before, during, and after this run?
Friday			
Saturday			
Sunday			

Take a moment to check in on your physical fatigue. Are you recovering from your workouts? Are you taking enough rest days to allow your body to recover? What has helped you to recover from a tough workout in the past?

Date:

My training goals for this week are:

I can mitigate obstacles this week by:

Day of the week	Distance/Speed	What was the purpose of this specific run?	How did I feel before, during, and after this run?
Monday			
Tuesday			
Wednesday			
Thursday			

Day of the week	Distance/Speed	What was the purpose of this specific run?	How did I feel before, during, and after this run?
Friday			
Saturday			
Sunday			

This week, I am most proud of myself for:

Date:

My training goals for this week are:

I can mitigate obstacles this week by:

Day of the week	Distance/Speed	What was the purpose of this specific run?	How did I feel before, during, and after this run?
Monday			
Tuesday			
Wednesday			
Thursday			

Day of the week	Distance/Speed	What was the purpose of this specific run?	How did I feel before, during, and after this run?
Friday			
Saturday			
Sunday			

Take a moment to rate your confidence level as well as your motivation level at this point in your training cycle.

Date:

My training goals for this week are:

I can mitigate obstacles this week by:

Day of the week	Distance/Speed	What was the purpose of this specific run?	How did I feel before, during, and after this run?
Monday			
Tuesday			
Wednesday			
Thursday			

Day of the week	Distance/Speed	What was the purpose of this specific run?	How did I feel before, during, and after this run?
Friday			
Saturday			
Sunday			

This week, I am most proud of myself for:

Date:

My training goals for this week are:

I can mitigate obstacles this week by:

Day of the week	Distance/Speed	What was the purpose of this specific run?	How did I feel before, during, and after this run?
Monday			
Tuesday			
Wednesday			
Thursday			

Day of the week	Distance/Speed	What was the purpose of this specific run?	How did I feel before, during, and after this run?
Friday			
Saturday			
Sunday			

This week, I am most proud of myself for:

Date:

My training goals for this week are:

I can mitigate obstacles this week by:

Day of the week	Distance/Speed	What was the purpose of this specific run?	How did I feel before, during, and after this run?
Monday			
Tuesday			
Wednesday			
Thursday			

Day of the week	Distance/Speed	What was the purpose of this specific run?	How did I feel before, during, and after this run?
Friday			
Saturday			
Sunday			

This week, I am most proud of myself for:

Date:

My training goals for this week are:

I can mitigate obstacles this week by:

Day of the week	Distance/Speed	What was the purpose of this specific run?	How did I feel before, during, and after this run?
Monday			
Tuesday			
Wednesday			
Thursday			

Day of the week	Distance/Speed	What was the purpose of this specific run?	How did I feel before, during, and after this run?
Friday			
Saturday			
Sunday			

This week, I am most proud of myself for:

Date:

My training goals for this week are:

I can mitigate obstacles this week by:

Day of the week	Distance/Speed	What was the purpose of this specific run?	How did I feel before, during, and after this run?
Monday			
Tuesday			
Wednesday			
Thursday			

Day of the week	Distance/Speed	What was the purpose of this specific run?	How did I feel before, during, and after this run?
Friday			
Saturday			
Sunday			

This week, I am most proud of myself for:

Date:

My training goals for this week are:

I can mitigate obstacles this week by:

Day of the week	Distance/Speed	What was the purpose of this specific run?	How did I feel before, during, and after this run?
Monday			
Tuesday			
Wednesday			
Thursday			

Day of the week	Distance/Speed	What was the purpose of this specific run?	How did I feel before, during, and after this run?
Friday			
Saturday			
Sunday			

How is your training fitting into your schedule? How might you make some changes to your schedule to improve your training? Consider times of the day that you feel more energetic and also consider training times in relation to meal times. Nutrition can propel runners towards success or hold them back.

Date:

My training goals for this week are:

I can mitigate obstacles this week by:

Day of the week	Distance/Speed	What was the purpose of this specific run?	How did I feel before, during, and after this run?
Monday			
Tuesday			
Wednesday			
Thursday			

Day of the week	Distance/Speed	What was the purpose of this specific run?	How did I feel before, during, and after this run?
Friday			
Saturday			
Sunday			

This week, I am most proud of myself for:

Date:

My training goals for this week are:

I can mitigate obstacles this week by:

Day of the week	Distance/Speed	What was the purpose of this specific run?	How did I feel before, during, and after this run?
Monday			
Tuesday			
Wednesday			
Thursday			

Day of the week	Distance/Speed	What was the purpose of this specific run?	How did I feel before, during, and after this run?
Friday			
Saturday			
Sunday			

This week, I am most proud of myself for:

Date:

My training goals for this week are:

I can mitigate obstacles this week by:

Day of the week	Distance/Speed	What was the purpose of this specific run?	How did I feel before, during, and after this run?
Monday			
Tuesday			
Wednesday			
Thursday			

Day of the week	Distance/Speed	What was the purpose of this specific run?	How did I feel before, during, and after this run?
Friday			
Saturday			
Sunday			

This week, I am most proud of myself for:

Date:

My training goals for this week are:

I can mitigate obstacles this week by:

Day of the week	Distance/Speed	What was the purpose of this specific run?	How did I feel before, during, and after this run?
Monday			
Tuesday			
Wednesday			
Thursday			

Day of the week	Distance/Speed	What was the purpose of this specific run?	How did I feel before, during, and after this run?
Friday			
Saturday			
Sunday			

This week, I am most proud of myself for:

9 SAMPLE TRAINING PLANS

This is a training workbook and is not designed to take the place of a training plan. Ideally, a training plan is tailored to meet the individual runner's goals and fitness level to ensure safety and success. If you do not have a training plan, there are many free generic training plans available online and affordable plans available from runnersworld.com. I have included some sample training plans in this chapter. These plans are examples of how runners with different goals could prepare for a variety of race distances. For a plan that is designed specifically for you to help you achieve your goals, I encourage that you reach out to a running trainer/ coach for support. These running professionals can work 1 to 1 with a runner and can provide group training services. I provide running training services including designing tailored training plans and utilizing coaching techniques that draw from sport psychology to promote mental training along with physical training. For more information about my services, please visit my website at ElevateRunning.org or reach out to me via email: ElevateRunningTraining@gmail.com.

Terms used in this chapter

- **Aerobic capacity:** during aerobic capacity training, the focus is increasing mileage and training is aimed at improving endurance.

- **Fartlek:** during a fartlek run, the runner varies their pace throughout their run and this variation can be based upon how the runner is feeling or on landmarks in their environment.

- **Intervals:** interval training involves fluctuating between high intensity and low intensity work periods.

- **Hill workouts:** hill workouts involve running hills and provide valuable strength training to runners. Hill workouts can be used to create more variety during training and help to prepare a runner for races that contain hills. Hill workouts can be added to any of the following sample training plans. When running hills, focus on your effort rather than your speed. Decrease hill training a couple of weeks before your race. I recommend that every runner include some hill workouts into their training regardless of whether or not the race that they are training for contains hills.

- **Acidosis threshold:** AT indicates the fastest pace that a runner can sustain at an aerobic level without utilizing significant anaerobic metabolism. AT training runs are designed to help raise a runner's AT pace allowing them to run a fast pace over long distances such as during a marathon. AT runs should be kept close to 10k race pace or 80-85% of max heart rate.

- **VO2 max:** VO2 max training is designed to increase aerobic power. VO2 max training pace is 95-100% of max heart rate or 20-25 seconds faster than 5k race pace.

- **Easy pace:** easy pace is approximately 70-75% of max heart rate. During easy runs, the runner should feel comfortable and should be able to maintain a conversation.

5k and 10k Sample Plans

The 5k and 10k plans below are based on time rather than distance. In other words, instead of listing mileage to complete on any given day, the plan lists minutes to complete. It is best to start any plan with some consistent running under your belt. All miles on these plans should be done at an easy pace unless noted otherwise. For some runners, this may mean alternating between running and walking to complete the duration listed on any given day. To create more diversity in these running plans, you can add additional training components such as fartlek runs or hill workouts depending on your current running fitness level.

16 Week 5k Sample Training Plan

Cycle 1: 4 weeks – Aerobic Capacity
Cycle 2: 4 weeks – Aerobic Capacity/Acidosis Threshold
Cycle 3: 4 weeks – Acidosis Threshold/VO2 Max
Cycle 4: 4 weeks – Acidosis Threshold/VO2 Max/Taper

Cycle 1: Aerobic Capacity

Week 1
M- Rest day
T- 25 minutes
W- 40 minutes
Th- 40 minutes
F- Rest day
S- 40 minutes
Su- 55 minutes
Total weekly training time: 200 minutes

Week 2
M- Rest day
T- 30 minutes
W- 40 minutes
Th- 45 minutes
F- Rest day
S- 40 minutes
Su- 60 minutes
Total weekly training time: 210 minutes

Week 3
M- Rest day
T- 30 minutes
W- 40 minutes
Th- 45 minutes

F- Rest day
S- 40 minutes
Su- 55 minutes
Total weekly training time: 210 minutes

Week 4
M- Rest day
T- 25 minutes
W- 25 minutes
Th- 25 minutes
F- Rest day
S- 30 minutes
Su- 35 minutes
Total weekly training time: 140 minutes

Cycle 2: Aerobic Capacity/Acidosis Threshold

Week 5
M- Rest day
T- 30 minutes
W- 40 minutes -AT run: 10 minutes warm up, 20 minutes AT pace, and 10 minutes cool down.
Th- 45 minutes
F- Rest day
S- 40 minutes -Fartlek run
Su- 55 minutes
Total weekly training time: 210 minutes

Week 6
M- Rest day
T- 35 minutes
W- 40 minutes -AT run: 10 minutes warm up, 20 minutes AT pace, and 10 minutes cool down.
Th- 45 minutes
F- Rest day
S- 40 minutes -Fartlek run
Su- 55 minutes
Total weekly training time: 220 minutes

Week 7
M- Rest day

T- 35 minutes
W- 40 minutes -AT run: 10 minutes warm up, 20 minutes AT pace, and 10 minutes cool down.
Th- 45 minutes
F- Rest day
S- 40 minutes -Fartlek run
Su- 60 minutes
Total weekly training time: 225 minutes

Week 8
M- Rest day
T- 25 minutes
W- 30 minutes -AT run: 10 minutes warm up, 10 minutes AT pace, and 10 minutes cool down.
Th- 30 minutes
F- Rest day
S- 30 minutes -Fartlek run
Su- 35 minutes
Total weekly training time: 150 minutes

Cycle 3: Acidosis Threshold/VO2 Max

Week 9
M- Rest day
T- 40 minutes -AT run: 10 minutes warm up, 20 minutes AT pace, and 10 minutes cool down.
W- 35 minutes
Th- 45 minutes -VO2 max run: 10 minutes warm up, 800 meter intervals at VO2 pace with 2 minutes easy pace between intervals, and 10 minutes cool down. If you continue to have energy, then continue intervals until you experience fatigue.
F- Rest day
S- 40 minutes
Su- 60 minutes
Total weekly training time: 225 minutes

Week 10
M- Rest day
T- 40 minutes -AT run: 10 minutes warm up, 20 minutes AT pace, and 10 minutes cool down.
W- 35 minutes

Th- 45 minutes -VO2 max run: 10 minutes warm up, 800 meter intervals at VO2 pace with 2 minutes easy pace between intervals, and 10 minutes cool down. If you continue to have energy, then continue intervals until you experience fatigue.
F- Rest day
S- 40 minutes
Su- 65 minutes
Total weekly training time: 230 minutes

Week 11
M- Rest day
T- 40 minutes -AT run: 10 minutes warm up, 20 minutes AT pace, and 10 minutes cool down.
W- 35 minutes
Th- 45 minutes -VO2 max run: 10 minutes warm up, 800 meter intervals at VO2 pace with 2 minutes easy pace between intervals, and 10 minutes cool down. If you continue to have energy, then continue intervals until you experience fatigue.
F- Rest day
S- 40 minutes
Su- 60 minutes
Total weekly training time: 225 minutes

Week 12
M- Rest day
T- 30 minutes -AT run: 10 minutes warm up, 10 minutes AT pace, and 10 minutes cool down.
W- 20 minutes
Th- 45 minutes -VO2 max run: 10 minutes warm up, 800 meter intervals at VO2 pace with 2 minutes easy pace between intervals, and 10 minutes cool down. If you continue to have energy, then continue intervals until you experience fatigue.
F- Rest day
S- 20 minutes
Su- 35 minutes
Total weekly training time: 150 minutes

Cycle 4: Acidosis Threshold/VO2 Max/Taper

Week 13
M- Rest day

T- 40 minutes -AT run: 10 minutes warm up, 20 minutes AT pace, and 10 minutes cool down.
W- 35 minutes
Th- 45 minutes -VO2 max run: 10 minutes warm up, 800 meter intervals at VO2 pace with 2 minutes easy pace between intervals, and 10 minutes cool down. If you continue to have energy, then continue intervals until you experience fatigue.
F- Rest day
S- 30 minutes
Su- 70 minutes
Total weekly training time: 225 minutes

Week 14
M- Rest day
T- 40 minutes -AT run: 10 minutes warm up, 20 minutes AT pace, and 10 minutes cool down.
W- 40 minutes
Th- 45 minutes -VO2 max run: 10 minutes warm up, 800 meter intervals at VO2 pace with 2 minutes easy pace between intervals, and 10 minutes cool down. If you continue to have energy, then continue intervals until you experience fatigue.
F- Rest day
S- 40 minutes
Su- 60 minutes
Total weekly training time: 230 minutes

Week 15
M- Rest day
T- 40 minutes -AT run: 10 minutes warm up, 20 minutes AT pace, and 10 minutes cool down.
W- 40 minutes
Th- 45 minutes -VO2 max run: 10 minutes warm up, 800 meter intervals at VO2 pace with 2 minutes easy pace between intervals, and 10 minutes cool down. If you continue to have energy, then continue intervals until you experience fatigue.
F- Rest day
S- 40 minutes
Su- 60 minutes
Total weekly training time: 230 minutes

Week 16

M- Rest day
T- 40 minutes -AT run: 10 minutes warm up, 20 minutes AT pace, and 10 minutes cool down.
W- 35 minutes
Th- 20 minutes
F- Rest day
S- 15 minutes
Su- 10 minutes
Total weekly training time: 130 minutes

5k Race Day!

16 Week 10k Sample Training Plan

Cycle 1: 4 weeks – Aerobic Capacity
Cycle 2: 4 weeks – Aerobic Capacity/Acidosis Threshold
Cycle 3: 4 weeks – Acidosis Threshold/VO2 Max
Cycle 4: 4 weeks – Acidosis Threshold/VO2 Max/Taper

Cycle 1: Aerobic Capacity

Week 1
M- Rest day
T- 35 minutes
W- 55 minutes
Th- 45 minutes
F- Rest day
S- 40 minutes
Su- 60 minutes
Total weekly training time: 235 minutes

Week 2
M- Rest day
T- 35 minutes
W- 55 minutes
Th- 45 minutes
F- Rest day
S- 40 minutes
Su- 65 minutes
Total weekly training time: 210 minutes

Week 3
M- Rest day
T- 35 minutes
W- 55 minutes
Th- 45 minutes
F- Rest day
S- 40 minutes
Su- 65 minutes
Total weekly training time: 240 minutes

Week 4
M- Rest day
T- 25 minutes
W- 35 minutes
Th- 25 minutes
F- Rest day
S- 30 minutes
Su- 45 minutes
Total weekly training time: 160 minutes

Cycle 2: Aerobic Capacity/Acidosis Threshold

Week 5
M- Rest day
T- 35 minutes
W- 55 minutes -AT run: 10 minutes warm up, 35 minutes AT pace, and 10 minutes cool down.
Th- 45 minutes
F- Rest day
S- 40 minutes
Su- 65 minutes
Total weekly training time: 240 minutes

Week 6
M- Rest day
T- 40 minutes
W- 55 minutes -AT run: 10 minutes warm up, 35 minutes AT pace, and 10 minutes cool down.
Th- 50 minutes

F- Rest day
S- 40 minutes
Su- 70 minutes
Total weekly training time: 255 minutes

Week 7
M- Rest day
T- 40 minutes
W- 55 minutes -AT run: 10 minutes warm up, 35 minutes AT pace, and 10 minutes cool down.
Th- 50 minutes
F- Rest day
S- 40 minutes
Su- 70 minutes
Total weekly training time: 255 minutes

Week 8
M- Rest day
T- 30 minutes
W- 45 minutes -AT run: 10 minutes warm up, 25 minutes AT pace, and 10 minutes cool down.
Th- 25 minutes
F- Rest day
S- 30 minutes
Su- 40 minutes
Total weekly training time: 170 minutes

Cycle 3: Acidosis Threshold/VO2 Max

Week 9
M- Rest day
T- 60 minutes -AT run: 10 minutes warm up, 35 minutes AT pace, and 10 minutes cool down.
W- 40 minutes
Th- 45 minutes -VO2 max run: 10 minutes warm up, 800 meter intervals at VO2 pace with 2 minutes easy pace between intervals, and 10 minutes cool down. If you continue to have energy, then continue intervals until you experience fatigue.
F- Rest day
S- 40 minutes
Su- 70 minutes

Total weekly training time: 255 minutes

Week 10
M- Rest day
T- 60 minutes -AT run: 10 minutes warm up, 35 minutes AT pace, and 10 minutes cool down.
W- 40 minutes
Th- 45 minutes -VO2 max run: 10 minutes warm up, 800 meter intervals at VO2 pace with 2 minutes easy pace between intervals, and 10 minutes cool down. If you continue to have energy, then continue intervals until you experience fatigue.
F- Rest day
S- 40 minutes
Su- 70 minutes
Total weekly training time: 255 minutes

Week 11
M- Rest day
T- 60 minutes -AT run: 10 minutes warm up, 35 minutes AT pace, and 10 minutes cool down.
W- 35 minutes
Th- 45 minutes -VO2 max run: 10 minutes warm up, 800 meter intervals at VO2 pace with 2 minutes easy pace between intervals, and 10 minutes cool down. If you continue to have energy, then continue intervals until you experience fatigue.
F- Rest day
S- 45 minutes
Su- 70 minutes
Total weekly training time: 255 minutes

Week 12
M- Rest day
T- 35 minutes -AT run: 10 minutes warm up, 15 minutes AT pace, and 10 minutes cool down.
W- 25 minutes
Th- 35 minutes -VO2 max run: 10 minutes warm up, 800 meter intervals at VO2 pace with 2 minutes easy pace between intervals, and 10 minutes cool down. If you continue to have energy, then continue intervals until you experience fatigue.
F- Rest day
S- 35 minutes

Su- 40 minutes
Total weekly training time: 170 minutes

Cycle 4: Acidosis Threshold/VO2 Max/Taper

Week 13
M- Rest day
T- 60 minutes -AT run: 10 minutes warm up, 35 minutes AT pace, and 10 minutes cool down.
W- 35 minutes
Th- 45 minutes -VO2 max run: 10 minutes warm up, 800 meter intervals at VO2 pace with 2 minutes easy pace between intervals, and 10 minutes cool down. If you continue to have energy, then continue intervals until you experience fatigue.
F- Rest day
S- 45 minutes
Su- 70 minutes
Total weekly training time: 255 minutes

Week 14
M- Rest day
T- 55 minutes -AT run: 10 minutes warm up, 30 minutes AT pace, and 10 minutes cool down.
W- 40 minutes
Th- 45 minutes -VO2 max run: 10 minutes warm up, 800 meter intervals at VO2 pace with 2 minutes easy pace between intervals, and 10 minutes cool down. If you continue to have energy, then continue intervals until you experience fatigue.
F- Rest day
S- 45 minutes
Su- 70 minutes
Total weekly training time: 255 minutes

Week 15
M- Rest day
T- 60 minutes -AT run: 10 minutes warm up, 35 minutes AT pace, and 10 minutes cool down.
W- 45 minutes
Th- 45 minutes -VO2 max run: 10 minutes warm up, 800 meter intervals at VO2 pace with 2 minutes easy pace between intervals,

and 10 minutes cool down. If you continue to have energy, then continue intervals until you experience fatigue.
F- Rest day
S- 45 minutes
Su- 60 minutes
Total weekly training time: 255 minutes

Week 16
M- Rest day
T- 55 minutes -AT run: 10 minutes warm up, 35 minutes AT pace, and 10 minutes cool down.
W- 35 minutes
Th- 20 minutes
F- Rest day
S- 15 minutes
Su- 10 minutes
Total weekly training time: 130 minutes

10k Race Day!

Half Marathon and Marathon Sample Plans

Unlike the 5k and 10k plans, the half marathon and marathon sample plans below are based on mileage rather than time. These plans should be used by runners who have been running consistently for some time with numerous long runs included in their training. It is very important to have solid regular mileage to build from especially with the marathon plan because it starts at a higher weekly mileage with longer long runs. These plans target aerobic capacity and acidosis threshold. As a runner continues to advance, VO2 max training should be incorporated. All miles on these plans should be done at an easy pace unless noted otherwise. To create more diversity in these running plans, you can add additional training components such as fartlek runs, hill workouts, or interval training depending on your current running fitness level.

20 Week Half Marathon Sample Training Plan

Cycle 1: 5 weeks – Aerobic Capacity

Cycle 2: 5 weeks – Aerobic Capacity
Cycle 3: 5 weeks – Aerobic Capacity/Acidosis Threshold
Cycle 4: 5 weeks – Aerobic Capacity/Acidosis Threshold/Taper

Cycle 1: Aerobic Capacity

Week 1
M- Rest day
T- 2 miles
W- 3 miles
Th- 3 miles
F- Rest day
S- 2 miles
Su- 5 miles
Total weekly mileage: 15 miles

Week 2
M- Rest day
T- 2 miles
W- 3 miles
Th- 3 miles
F- Rest day
S- 2 miles
Su- 6 miles
Total weekly mileage: 16 miles

Week 3
M- Rest day
T- 3 miles
W- 3 miles
Th- 3 miles
F- Rest day
S- 3 miles
Su- 7 miles
Total weekly mileage: 19 miles

Week 4
M- Rest day
T- 3 miles
W- 3 miles
Th- 3 miles

F- Rest day
S- 3 miles
Su- 7 miles
Total weekly mileage: 19 miles

Week 5
M- Rest day
T- 2 miles
W- 3 miles
Th- 3 miles
F- Rest day
S- 2 miles
Su- 3 miles
Total weekly mileage: 13 miles

Cycle 2: Aerobic Capacity

Week 6
M- Rest day
T- 3 miles
W- 3 miles
Th- 4 miles
F- Rest day
S- 3 miles
Su- 7 miles
Total weekly mileage: 20 miles

Week 7
M- Rest day
T- 3 miles
W- 3 miles
Th- 4 miles
F- Rest day
S- 3 miles
Su- 7 miles
Total weekly mileage: 20 miles

Week 8
M- Rest day
T- 4 miles
W- 5 miles

Th- 4 miles
F- Rest day
S- 3 miles
Su- 8 miles
Total weekly mileage: 24 miles

Week 9
M- Rest day
T- 4 miles
W- 5 miles
Th- 4 miles
F- Rest day
S- 3 miles
Su- 8 miles
Total weekly mileage: 24 miles

Week 10
M- Rest day
T- 2 miles
W- 3 miles
Th- 3 miles
F- Rest day
S- 2 miles
Su- 6 miles
Total weekly mileage: 16 miles

Cycle 3: Aerobic Capacity/Acidosis Threshold

Week 11
M- Rest day
T- 4 miles
W- 4 miles -AT run: 10 min warm up and 10 min cool down with the mid-section of the run kept at AT pace
Th- 4 miles
F- Rest day
S- 4 miles
Su- 8 miles
Total weekly mileage: 24 miles

Week 12
M- Rest day

T- 4 miles
W- 4 miles -AT run: 10 min warm up and 10 min cool down with the mid-section of the run kept at AT pace
Th- 4 miles
F- Rest day
S- 3 miles
Su- 9 miles
Total weekly mileage: 24 miles

Week 13
M- Rest day
T- 4 miles
W- 5 miles -AT run: 10 min warm up and 10 min cool down with the mid-section of the run kept at AT pace
Th- 5 miles
F- Rest day
S- 4 miles
Su- 10 miles
Total weekly mileage: 28 miles

Week 14
M- Rest day
T- 4 miles
W- 5 miles -AT run: 10 min warm up and 10 min cool down with the mid-section of the run kept at AT pace
Th- 4 miles
F- Rest day
S- 4 miles
Su- 11 miles
Total weekly mileage: 28 miles

Week 15
M- Rest day
T- 3 miles
W- 3 miles -AT run: 10 min warm up and 10 min cool down with the mid-section of the run kept at AT pace
Th- 3 miles
F- Rest day
S- 3 miles
Su- 7 miles
Total weekly mileage: 19 miles

Cycle 4: Aerobic Capacity/Acidosis Threshold

Week 16
M- Rest day
T- 4 miles
W- 5 miles -AT run: 10 min warm up and 10 min cool down with the mid-section of the run kept at AT pace
Th- 4 miles
F- Rest day
S- 4 miles
Su- 12 miles
Total weekly mileage: 28 miles

Week 17
M- Rest day
T- 4 miles
W- 5 miles -AT run: 10 min warm up and 10 min cool down with the mid-section of the run kept at AT pace
Th- 4 miles
F- Rest day
S- 3 miles
Su- 13 miles
Total weekly mileage: 28 miles

Week 18
M- Rest day
T- 4 miles
W- 5 miles -AT run: 10 min warm up and 10 min cool down with the mid-section of the run kept at AT pace
Th- 4 miles
F- Rest day
S- 4 miles
Su- 12 miles
Total weekly mileage: 28 miles

Week 19
M- Rest day
T- 4 miles

W- 4 miles -AT run: 10 min warm up and 10 min cool down with the mid-section of the run kept at AT pace
Th- 3 miles
F- Rest day
S- 3 miles
Su- 11 miles
Total weekly mileage: 25 miles

Week 20
M- Rest day
T- 4 miles
W- 3 miles
Th- 3 miles
F- Rest day
S- 2 miles
Su-1 miles
Total weekly mileage: 13 miles

Half Marathon Race Day!

20 Week Marathon Sample Training Plan

Cycle 1: 5 weeks – Aerobic Capacity
Cycle 2: 5 weeks – Aerobic Capacity
Cycle 3: 5 weeks – Aerobic Capacity/Acidosis Threshold
Cycle 4: 5 weeks – Aerobic Capacity/Acidosis Threshold/Taper

Cycle 1: Aerobic Capacity

Week 1
M- Rest day
T- 4 miles
W- 5 miles
Th- 4 miles
F- 5 miles
S- 4 miles
Su- 13 miles
Total weekly mileage: 35 miles

Week 2

M- Rest day
T- 4 miles
W- 5 miles
Th- 5 miles
F- 5 miles
S- 4 miles
Su- 14 miles
Total weekly mileage: 36 miles

Week 3
M- Rest day
T- 4 miles
W- 5 miles
Th- 5 miles
F- 5 miles
S- 4 miles
Su- 14 miles
Total weekly mileage: 36 miles

Week 4
M- Rest day
T- 4 miles
W- 5 miles
Th- 5 miles
F- 5 miles
S- 4 miles
Su- 15 miles
Total weekly mileage: 37 miles

Week 5
M- Rest day
T- 3 miles
W- 4 miles
Th- 3 miles
F- 4 miles
S- 3 miles
Su- 8 miles
Total weekly mileage: 25 miles

Cycle 2: Aerobic Capacity

Week 6
M- Rest day
T- 4 miles
W- 5 miles
Th- 4 miles
F- 5 miles
S- 3 miles
Su- 16 miles
Total weekly mileage: 37 miles

Week 7
M- Rest day
T- 4 miles
W- 5 miles
Th- 4 miles
F- 5 miles
S- 3 miles
Su- 17 miles
Total weekly mileage: 38 miles

Week 8
M- Rest day
T- 4 miles
W- 5 miles
Th- 4 miles
F- 5 miles
S- 3 miles
Su- 17 miles
Total weekly mileage: 38 miles

Week 9
M- Rest day
T- 4 miles
W- 5 miles
Th- 4 miles
F- 5 miles
S- 3 miles
Su- 18 miles
Total weekly mileage: 39 miles

Week 10

M- Rest day
T- 3 miles
W- 4 miles
Th- 3 miles
F- 4 miles
S- 3 miles
Su- 10 miles
Total weekly mileage: 27 miles

Cycle 3: Aerobic Capacity/Acidosis Threshold

Week 11
M- Rest day
T- 4 miles
W- 5 miles
Th- 4 miles
F- 5 miles
S- 3 miles
Su- 19 miles
Total weekly mileage: 40 miles

Week 12
M- Rest day
T- 5 miles
W- 5 miles -AT run: 10 min warm up and 10 min cool down with the mid-section of the run kept at AT pace
Th- 5 miles
F- 5 miles
S- 4 miles
Su- 16 miles
Total weekly mileage: 40 miles

Week 13
M- Rest day
T- 4 miles
W- 6 miles
Th- 6 miles
F- 5 miles
S- 4 miles
Su- 19 miles
Total weekly mileage: 42 miles

Week 14
M- Rest day
T- 5 miles
W- 6 miles -AT run: 10 min warm up and 10 min cool down with the mid-section of the run kept at AT pace
Th- 6 miles
F- 5 miles
S- 5 miles
Su- 14 miles
Total weekly mileage: 41 miles

Week 15
M- Rest day
T- 3 miles
W- 5 miles -AT run: 10 min warm up and 10 min cool down with the mid-section of the run kept at AT pace
Th- 5 miles
F- 4 miles
S- 3 miles
Su- 10 miles
Total weekly mileage: 30 miles

Cycle 4: Aerobic Capacity/Acidosis Threshold

Week 16
M- Rest day
T- 4 miles
W- 5 miles
Th- 6 miles
F- 5 miles
S- 4 miles
Su- 17 miles
Total weekly mileage: 43 miles

Week 17
M- Rest day
T- 4 miles
W- 5 miles -AT run: 10 min warm up and 10 min cool down with the mid-section of the run kept at AT pace

Th- 4 miles
F- 5 miles
S- 3 miles
Su- 14 miles
Total weekly mileage: 44 miles

Week 18
M- Rest day
T- 4 miles
W- 5 miles
Th- 6 miles
F- 5 miles
S- 4 miles
Su- 16 miles
Total weekly mileage: 45 miles

Week 19
M- Rest day
T- 4 miles
W- 5 miles -AT run: 10 min warm up and 10 min cool down with the mid-section of the run kept at AT pace
Th- 4 miles
F- 5 miles
S- 4 miles
Su- 15 miles
Total weekly mileage: 42 miles

Week 20
M- Rest day
T- 4 miles
W- 3 miles
Th- 3 miles
F- Rest day
S- 2 miles
Su- 1 miles
Total weekly mileage: 13 miles

Marathon Race Day!

ABOUT THE AUTHOR

Julia is a certified running trainer, certified personal trainer, certified yoga teacher, and licensed marriage and family therapist. She is a passionate marathon runner and began offering running training services in March 2018. She has obtained undergraduate and graduate degrees in psychology and uses principles from sport psychology to inform her running training services.

In February 2019, Julia founded Elevate Running, a business providing running coaching that addresses both mental & physical training to enhance performance. For information about Elevate Running and additional running resources, please visit ElevateRunning.org

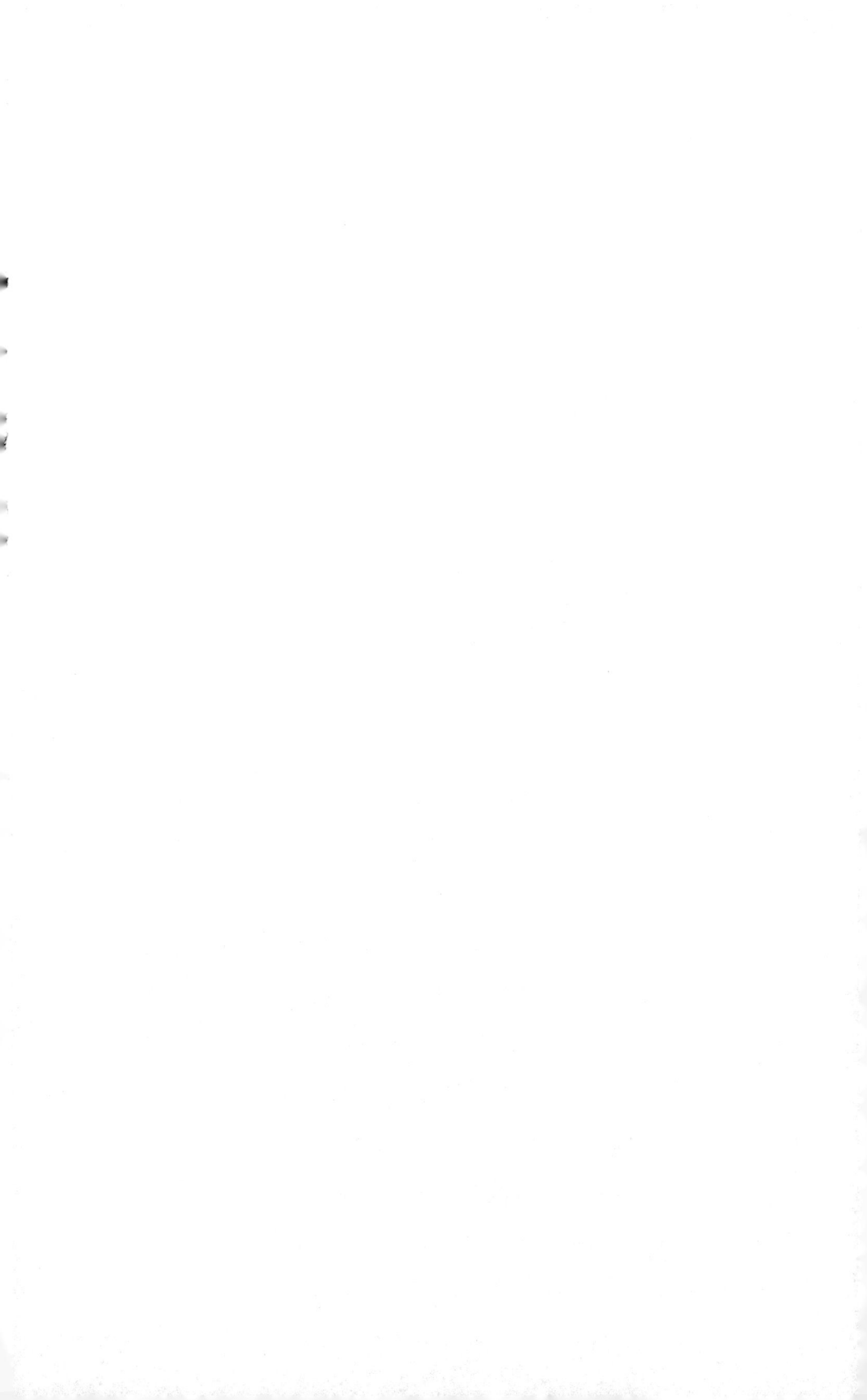

Made in the USA
Lexington, KY
07 June 2019